SODIUM BICARBONATE

NATURE'S UNIQUE FIRST AID REMEDY

DR. MARK SIRCUS

COVER DESIGNER: Jeannie Tudor
EDITOR: Erica Shur
TYPESETTER: Gary A. Rosenberg

The information and advice contained in this book are based upon the research and the personal and professional experiences of the author. They are not intended as a substitute for consulting with a health care professional. The publisher and author are not responsible for any adverse effects or consequences resulting from the use of any of the suggestions, preparations, or procedures discussed in this book. All matters pertaining to your physical health should be supervised by a health care professional. It is a sign of wisdom, not cowardice, to seek a second or third opinion.

Square One Publishers
115 Herricks Road
Garden City Park, NY 11040
(516) 535-2010 • (877) 900-BOOK
www.squareonepublishers.com

Library of Congress Cataloging-in-Publication Data
Sircus, Mark.
  Sodium bicarbonate : nature's unique first aid remedy / Dr. Mark Sircus.
      pages cm
  Includes bibliographical references and index.
  ISBN 978-0-7570-0394-3
  1. Sodium bicarbonate—Therapeutic use. 2. Traditional medicine. I. Title.
  TP245.S7S54 2014
  661'.323--dc23
                              2014006254

Printed in the United States of America

10   9   8   7   6   5   4   3

Contents

To Vernon Johnston

Introduction

This is the first medical review of sodium bicarbonate (baking soda) in the history of medicine and it will change the way you think about baking soda, change the way we practice medicine and change the way we take care of our children. Our lives are made easier by sodium bicarbonate for there are hundreds of uses for it. It helps us clean up messes around the house as well as messes inside our bodies.

When Hippocrates said in 400 BC, "Let food be thy medicine," he did not dream that individual vitamins, minerals, and even enzymes could be taken in concentrated form. Almost twenty-five hundred years later, the best emergency room and intensive care doctors use concentrated nutritional medicine to save lives every day, including baking soda. Sodium bicarbonate is a world class emergency room and intensive care medicine used every day to save lives.

Until now you could only find books about the household use baking soda so its use as a medicine has been shrouded in mystery. No longer! Sodium bicarbonate, known chemically as $NaHCO_3$, is a form of salt that has many names, including baking soda, bread soda, and bicarbonate of soda. It is found in nature in a crystalline form, which may be processed into a fine powder. It has long been used for a variety of medicinal purposes, but is not a pharmaceutical drug.

Sodium bicarbonate is the time honored method to 'speed up' the return of the body's bicarbonate levels to normal. Bicarbonate is the ion normally responsible for alkalinity, or the capacity of water to neutralize acids or resist changes in pH. Sodium bicarbonate neutralizes acid and protects digestive enzymes. Sodium bicarbonate happens to be one of our most useful medicines treating as it does basic human physiology.

Sodium bicarbonate is only classified as a medicine if injected or administered intravenously. Otherwise, it is a legal food item that anyone can buy in most supermarkets and pharmacies around the world. It is totally safe because not only does the body need it but it also produces it in the stomach, pancreas and kidneys.

Sodium bicarbonate is nutritional but is one of the most concentrated effective medicines in the world. Its ranges of effects are profound. It has blood vessel dilating action (vasodilator), increases blood fluidity, facilitates blood flow delivery as well as assisting oxygen dissociation from hemoglobin—thus more oxygen flows to the capillaries and cells. Through the "Bohr Effect" more oxygen is released from hemoglobin.

Bicarbonate also has strong anti-inflammatory action, helps with detoxification and neutralization of toxic substances of all kinds offering strong and almost instantaneous shifts in pH. Pharmaceutical companies can charge all they want, and they do for their dangerous ineffective medicines. But even in the wildest dreams of a pharmaceutical executive do visions come for a drug they might fabricate that would match the fantastic medicinal properties of simple inexpensive baking soda.

The pH of the blood is the most important factor to determine the state of the microorganisms in the blood.

Sodium bicarbonate acts as a powerful, natural and safe antifungal agent, which when combined with iodine, covers the entire spectrum of microbial organisms. The efficacy of sodium bicarbonate against certain bacteria and fungi has been documented but its role as a disinfectant against viruses is not generally known. Sodium bicarbonate at concentrations of 5 percent and above was found to be effective with 99.99 percent reduction of viral titers on food contact surfaces within a contact time of one minute.[1]

Safe Medicine for Nuclear Contamination

There is an extraordinary reason why everyone needs to understand and use baking soda. The radiation from Fukushima is relentless and getting worse spreading far and wide on our beautiful planet and one of the most potent uses of sodium bicarbonate is as an antidote for radiation exposure.

It is a crying shame what we have done to ourselves and our children by allowing nuclear power, nuclear weapons and depleted uranium armaments. As we shall see in this book baking soda is one of the best antidotes for radiation poisoning. One can easily and cheaply take it orally or pile it into ones baths and this does offer a good measure of protection. It's the same reason why sodium bicarbonate is an excellent treatment for cancer. Research concludes that sodium bicarbonate increases tumor pH and inhibits spontaneous metastases.

Radiation exposure and increased incidences of cancer are tied mathematically to each other so whatever is good for treating cancer is effective for treating radiation exposure. My writings and work with sodium bicarbonate began when I found out that bicarbonate was used by the Army for uranium exposure to protect the kidneys and after learning about Dr. Tullio Simoncini and his work with sodium bicarbonate, cancer and its use as a fungicide to irradiate Candida infections.

The title of my original writings on bicarbonate was *Rich Man's Poor Man's Cancer Treatment* and it is that without doubt. This book though is not saying that sodium bicarbonate is the cure to cancer but it is saying that almost every cancer patient should be taking it increasing substantially one's chance of becoming a cancer survivor. This is more than important in a world where one out of every two people will sooner or later get cancer and the numbers seem destined to only get worse.

Nutritional Medicine

Sodium bicarbonate is not a pharmaceutical drug it is a nutrient the body needs for survival every day. Literally thousands of studies have uncovered a clear and distinct relationship between vital nutrients and cancer. One influential study (Ramesha et al. 1990) provides a powerful example. A powerful carcinogen known as DMBA was given to a group of female rats. Then the rats were given none, one of four, two of four, three of four, or all of four nutrients: the minerals selenium and magnesium, and vitamins C and A.

When no nutrients were administered, all of the rats developed breast cancer. When one of the nutrients was given, 46.4 to 57.1 percent of the rats developed tumors, depending on the nutrient. When two of the nutrients were given in combination, the tumor incidence decreased to 29.9 to 34.6 percent, depending on which nutrients were used in combination. Administration of nutrients in groups of threes resulted in further reduction of tumor incidences coming down to somewhere between 16 to 23.1 percent. And when all four nutrients were given together, tumor incidence dropped to 12 percent. Human DNA is 99 percent identical to that of rats.

Natural Cancer Medicine

This book is about the application of the least expensive, safest and perhaps most effective cancer medicine there is, and that is the primary reason so many people have been interested in my writings and research on sodium bicarbonate.

Simple baking soda is a prime, in fact second most important of my Natural Allopathic Medicine protocol for cancer (which includes the nutrients in the above study) holding down the number two spot coming right after magnesium. My approach to cancer as well as all other diseases is a protocol approach, which includes other powerful non-toxic substances like glutathione, iodine, selenium, vitamin C, light and heat, as well as other substances that are prioritized to yield a powerful yet all natural treatment for cancer.

Most of us were amazed to find out that there is an oncologist in Rome, Dr. Tullio Simoncini destroying cancer tumors with sodium bicarbonate. Sodium bicarbonate is safe, extremely inexpensive and effective when it comes to cancer tissues. It is irresistible cyanide to cancer cells. It hits the cancer cells with a shock wave of alkalinity, which allows much more oxygen into the cancer cells than they can tolerate. Cancer cells cannot survive in the presence of high levels of oxygen. Sodium bicarbonate is a killer of tumors, safer and more effective than anything else. That does not mean that every single patient who uses bicarbonate is going to be saved but they certainly will be helped.

Treatment takes only as few weeks too several months. Even if a person does not survive their cancer the bicarbonate will bring comfort and reduction of pain. When successful follow up treatments, are then, highly recommended. Over the long term health habit changes are paramount. Certain substances, like magnesium, bicarbonate, iodine and selenium are mineral medicines we all should be taking for life. All of our bodies are under stresses never before faced across a broad front of radiation exposures (medical testing), chemical and heavy metal exposure, and the tremendous explosion of microwave transmission. We need these minerals just like plants do.

It All Started Here

Dr. Tullio Simoncini tells us of his early experience with bicarbonate. "One of the first patients I treated was an 11-year-old child, a case which immediately indicated that I was on the right track. The child arrived in a coma at the paediatrichaematology ward around 11:30 in the morning, with a clinical history of leukemia. Because of the child's disease he had been taken from a small town in Sicily to Rome, through the universities of Palermo and Naples, where he underwent several chemotherapy sessions. His desperate mother told me that she had been unable to speak with the child for 15 days; that is, since the child had been on his journey through the various hospitals. She said she would have given the world to hear her son's voice once again before he died."

"As I was of the opinion that the child was comatose both because of the proliferation of fungal colonies in the brain and because of the toxicity of the therapies that had been performed on him, I concluded that if I could destroy the colonies with sodium bicarbonate salts and at the same time nourish and detoxify the brain with glucose administered intravenously, I could hope for a regression of the symptoms. And so it was. After a continuous intravenous infusion of bicarbonate and glucose solutions, at around 7 pm, when I returned to the university, I found the child speaking with his mother, who was in tears," said Dr. Simoncini.

There is an amazing amount of materials on sodium bicarbonate and baking soda on the Internet and I am responsible for much of it over the years. Hard not to be moved by such testimonials but many discount such information as unscientific yet there is nothing unscientific about sodium bicarbonate because we are talking basic chemistry.

In this book most of the testimonials are personal accounts but throughout the book I share clinical experience of professionals as well as the conclusions of studies and reports.

Natural Chemotherapy

Sodium bicarbonate cancer treatment focuses on delivering natural chemotherapy in a way that effectively kills cancer cells while dramatically reducing the brutal side effects and costs experienced with standard chemotherapy treatments. Everyone should know about this and it is a betrayal of our humanity that most people still do not know. Losing the benefits and comfort that sodium bicarbonate (and magnesium bicarbonate and potassium bicarbonate and even calcium bicarbonate can bring).

One pound of sodium bicarbonate costs only a few dollars at the supermarket. If you live in the States you can get fifty pounds for fifty dollars of high grade medicine that you can drink or put in your bathtub for the quickest, safest and certainly least expensive anticancer treatment available anywhere for any price.

For less than a dinner at a restaurant one has a nothing-to-lose-every-thing-to-gain-cancer-treatment. Sodium bicarbonate is an effective, safe and rapid acting anti-tumor agent. It is a necessary cancer medicine and oncologists have secretly been using it for decades to protect their patients from the deadly chemo chemicals they use.

Oncologist's Secret Weapon

Sodium bicarbonate is used prior to, during, and after application of chemotherapy.[2] Studies have already shown how manipulation of tumor pH with sodium bicarbonate enhances chemotherapy[3] pointing to the appropriateness of using bicarbonate as a principle medicinal substance with the potential of curing people of their cancers.

Since the very beginning sodium bicarbonate has been used with the premier chemotherapy agent made from mustard gas. Mechlorethamine also known as chlormethine, mustine, nitrogen mustard and HN_2 and sold under the brand name Mustargen was the prototype anticancer chemotherapeutic drug. Use of mechlorethamine gave birth to the field of anticancer chemotherapy. Without baking soda orthodox oncology would never have been able to establish itself for all their patients would probably have died too quickly.

You will also be given lots of fluids (as a drip) and a drug called mesna with your cyclophosphamide to help prevent bladder irritation. Sodium bicarbonate will be given to you—usually as a drip—before and during your methotrexate treatment, to help protect your kidneys.[4]

These chemo drugs are an analogue of mustard gas and were derived from chemical warfare research. Instructions for their use include: Dilute well with rapidly running IVF flush solution. After infusion is complete, give brisk bolus approx. 200 cc IVF to flush veins. The basic substances used in IVF flushes are sodium thiosulfate[5] and sodium bicarbonate. Without the bicarbonate and thiosulfate buffers patients would quickly succumb to the chemo poisons. It's a picture right out of hell using mustard gas instead of something vastly safer.

Everyone who chooses highly toxic and dangerous chemotherapy should be advised that science indicates that it might be the sodium bicarbonate that's doing the helping and not the poisons. Wouldn't it be sickening to think that patients had to take a pile of poison just to get their simple, inexpensive and safe bicarbonate treatments? The story and history of chemotherapy would have been a lot worse if sodium bicarbonate was not already in wide use for cancer patients taking chemotherapy.

1. *Bicarbonate Fundamentals*

When we are hovering close to death, bicarbonate will do the job it is meant to do. Sodium bicarbonate is a mainstream emergency room intensive care medicine. It is fast-acting, safe, concentrated, injectable nutritional medicine. When all else fails sodium bicarbonate can save the day. Emergency room and intensive care medicine would be severely handicapped if there was no sodium bicarbonate and already extremely dangerous chemotherapy would be even more deadly without bicarbonate used as a buffer when the chemical chemo poisons are pumped in.

Sodium bicarbonate delivers lifesaving healing power. It can be taken orally, used transdermally, through nebulization, or administered intravenously or by injection by a doctor or a nurse in more desperate medical situations.

If you want to see how fast a person can hit the floor during chemotherapy just forget to mix in the bicarbonate and get out your stopwatch. Most doctors are not aware that sodium bicarbonate is used routinely to keep the toxicity of chemotherapy agents and radiation from killing people or from destroying their kidneys.

Sodium bicarbonate acts as a natural and safe antifungal agent, which when combined with iodine, covers the entire spectrum of microbial organisms. The efficacy of sodium bicarbonate against certain bacteria and fungi has been documented but its role as a disinfectant against viruses is not generally known. Sodium bicarbonate at concentrations of 5 percent and above was found to be effective with 99.99 percent reduction of viral titers on food contact surfaces within a contact time of one minute.[1]

Taking sodium bicarbonate orally or bathing in a tub saturated with it results in a shift of the body's pH to less acidic and more alkaline. That's because baking soda is an electron donor. As the pH rises, so does cellular voltage and cellular oxygen levels.

We increase cell voltage, raise energy and performance levels of cellular activity when we supplement with sodium bicarbonate, which has long been known as an excellent medicine for the kidneys, and dialysis units use bicarbonate regularly but they, like everyone else, don't want to brag about it. Professionals do not want to get caught with their pants down using something as simple, cheap and non-pharmaceutical as baking soda.

The story of sodium bicarbonate is a long one for it has been in use as a medicine for over 150 years. Everyone knows of the Arm and Hammer brand but few doctors or people understand why it is such an excellent medicine. The secret of sodium bicarbonate is in the bicarbonate ion. It's not about sodium!

Sodium bicarbonate is one of the most potent medicines emergency room and intensive care doctors have because the bicarbonate ion is able to explode onto the scene of cell physiology almost instantly. The body does not usually need the extra sodium but the body is always hungry for bicarbonate unless you live in some pristine valley eating perfect food drinking pure water.

North Americans use a billion pounds of sodium bicarbonate each year, according to Bryan Thomlison, director of public affairs for Church and Dwight, the world's major manufacturer of sodium bicarbonate located in Princeton, N.J. "Usage is up 3 percent per year. That's twice as fast as the population growth."

The public is waking up to how useful sodium bicarbonate is. Baking soda is moving out of the refrigerator and into an amazing array of commercial products from shampoo to industrial cleansers, tooth paste and now into cancer and other chronic disease treatments, where there is a desperate need for its almost magical chemistry balancing act.

The clear message of this book is that there is no reason to not self-medicate with bicarbonate in cancer and most other clinical situations.

How Does Sodium Bicarbonate Affect The Body?

It is established that sodium bicarbonate does not raise blood pressure like common table salt does. When one consumes salt there are no minerals left and that makes all the difference in terms of blood pressure regulation. When one uses what are considered whole or unprocessed salts again we do not see the rise in blood pressure that we do with processed salt because all the mineral necessary for life are present.

Bicarbonate has a commanding power over a central biological axis of life—the pH buffer system and thus the relative alkalinity of the body's tissues. Every biochemical reaction is pH sensitive with enzymes being especially sensitive. Your pH level influences the activity of every metabolic function that takes place in your body. pH is behind the body's electrical system and intracellular activity as well as the way it utilizes enzymes, minerals, and vitamins.

All cancer sufferers, and in fact every chronic disease patient, should hold clearly in mind that pH is a regulatory authority that controls most cellular processes. The pH balance of the human bloodstream is recognized by medical physiology texts as one of the most important biochemical balances.

Several weeks ago, I purchased your book about Sodium Bicarbonate. *It changed my life.* I believe that God is working through you and your staff to spread the word about the body's natural ability to heal, given the right elements. Thank you! I've been reading your newsletter for some time now, and happened to see your book about baking soda. We don't have a lot of money, but I felt that your research might help me. Sure enough I can tell you that within the week following reading your book—and practicing what you preach—I have been practically hive—urticaria free.

I started with straight baking soda and water. Yuck! I could hardly make myself do it. But I was going for the pH balance you talked about. I read more about the different oral combinations and decided to try the maple syrup and baking soda, 3:1. It worked great and tasted great too. I couldn't believe I could eat that much sugar!

Right now I'm smiling and feeling great. My mood is good, my energy is way up and most important the swellings and itching are gone. My hair is growing back thicker. My skin looks great. I'm not tired all the time. I can't believe the difference in my health. Praise God for his goodness in inspiring your work.

I've recently added Nascent Iodine after reading some tips of yours. I was indeed deficient and that seems to be adding to the overall good effects. My children are benefiting from this research as well. I'm so happy to find alternatives to mainstream medicine.

L C, Delaware, United States

Our body pH is important because pH controls the speed of our body's biochemical reactions. It does this by controlling the speed of enzyme activity as well as the speed that electricity moves through our body—the higher (more alkaline) the pH of a substance or solution, the more electrical resistance that substance or solution holds.

Body pH level changes are intense in the profoundness of their biological effects. Even genes directly experience external pH. Important changes in pH may not only affect the shape of an enzyme but it may also change the shape or charge properties of the substrate.[2] When pH is too low, meaning the body is overly acidic, either the substrate cannot bind to the active site or it cannot undergo catalysis. Increased oxidative stress, which correlates almost exponentially with pH changes into the acidic, is especially dangerous to the mitochondria, which suffer the greatest under oxidative duress. Epigenetics, which may now have begun eclipsing traditional genetics, commonly describes how factors such as diet and smoking, rather than inheritance, influence how genes behave.

Each enzyme works within quite a small pH range. There is a pH at which its activity is greatest (the optimal pH). This is because changes in pH can make and break intra- and intermolecular bonds, changing the shape of the enzyme and, therefore, its effectiveness.

Making Patients Feel Better

"I have used intravenous sodium bicarbonate therapy mostly as a naturopathic treatment for patients who consistently react to allergens or that have chemical sensitivities. This is a great therapy during the Vancouver allergy seasons of spring and fall. The alkalinizing sodium bicarbonate IV can often immediately stop an allergic reaction, or asthmatic attack, since such reactions cannot persist in an alkaline environment. Some of my patients also get benefit from taking an alkalinizing drink every night to reduce their chemical sensitivity symptoms," writes Dr Eric Chan. "All of my Vancouver and Richmond patients have tolerated this therapy markedly well."

"Uniformly, in ill patients, increasing the alkaline buffer of the tissues makes patients feel better. As mentioned above, this is particularly true in chemically sensitive patients, and can actually be a 'cure' in the sense that we are increasing the body's ability to react in a healthy way to noxious stimuli. If I use the intravenous sodium bicarbonate in such patients, it is usually given twice a week for a period of 4 to 5 weeks. Sodium bicarbonate is a very effective way of directly improving cellular health by making the tissue more alkaline," concludes Dr. Chan.

Sodium bicarbonate loading and continuous infusion was associated with a lower incidence of acute renal dysfunction in cardiac surgical patients undergoing cardiopulmonary bypass.[3]

Sodium bicarbonate is the time honored method to "speed up" the return of the body's bicarbonate levels to normal. Bicarbonate is inorganic, very alkaline and like other mineral type substances supports an extensive list of biological functions. Sodium bicarbonate happens to be one of our most useful medicines because bicarbonate physiology is fundamental to life and health. So helpful and elementary it's even instrumental in helping sperm swim up and enter the cervical canal.[4]

Useful in Most Medical Situations

Sodium bicarbonate (baking soda) is used as an ingredient in some mouth-washes. It works as a mechanical cleanser on the teeth and gums, neutral-izes the production of acid in the mouth, and is also used as an antiseptic to help prevent infections occurring. Antiseptics are antimicrobial sub-stances that are applied to living tissue/skin to reduce the possibility of infection, sepsis, or putrefaction. Antiseptics are generally distinguished from antibiotics by their ability to be transported through the lymphatic sys-tem to destroy bacteria within the body, and from disinfectants, which destroy microorganisms found on non-living objects. A statistically signifi-cant ($p < 0.05$) reduction in numbers of mutans streptococci is seen when bicarbonate is used for oral care.

Some antiseptics are true germicides, capable of destroying microbes (bacteriocidal), whilst others are bacteriostatic and only prevent or inhibit their growth. Antibacterials are antiseptics that have the proven ability to act against bacteria especially if they target systems which kill only bacteria. Microbicides which kill virus particles are called viricides or antivirals.

In a 1947 issue of *British Medical Journal*, Dr. Hedda Gorz (Polish Hospi-tal, Storrington) writes:

> During the insurrection in Warsaw we were very short of all drugs, par-ticularly of antiseptics. We used a solution of 5 percent sodium bicarbon-ate for dressing of wounds and for operations. The results appeared to be excellent. All of us were greatly satisfied of obtained results and I used it afterwards in my further practice. For two months the patients were treated in cellars and other very inadequate conditions without water or drugs. Working in such terrible conditions—field hospitals set in cellars and underground shelters—all patients whose wounds were open, dirty, and contaminated with dust of the bombed houses were only treated with the 5 percent solution of sodium bicarbonate, the only

one obtainable there. All heavy cases in badly ventilated cellars became tolerable after dressing with this solution, even open lung wounds notorious for their fetor as well known to every surgeon.

Bicarbonate Lotions

You can also or make a paste of baking soda and water (3 parts baking soda to 1 part water) and apply directly to more localized rashes and irritations. When you use this method the water evaporates quite quickly leaving a layer of baking soda on the skin. Sodium bicarbonate is a therapeutic drug for vertigo.[5] The neurological story on sodium bicarbonate is an interesting one. For example, if I accidentally take any aspartame products, now commonly found hidden in many gums and even children's supplements (such as Flintstones vitamins), the urinary pH will go immediately acid to urinary pH of 5.5 or below.

The neurological system controls the body's pH, much like a thermometer. Aspartame in presences of the body's enzymes breaks down into methanol and then formaldehyde. When this happens, the body becomes acid quite quickly and then the neurological system burns itself up, and hence the immune system and the homeostatic mechanism which helps maintain the body's system.

As a simple antidote one can take baking soda to protect oneself from neurological damage. In fact the brain's pH is relatively acid due to most of the oxygen of the body, on a per weight basis, is consumed by the brain and hence it is relatively sensitive to damage.

Biological Treatments for Autism and PDD

One mother wrote, "It worked so well for both of my children that the die-off was an uneventful experience, even though they both had very high levels of yeast." The restoring of acid/alkaline balance also relieves many allergies. "These children also had grave disturbances in electrolyte chemistry, and tended to be acidotic (low CO). The data that unfolded was fascinating and clearly earmarked the acidosis and hypoxic state (low serum bicarbonate = low O_2 levels). Potassium bicarbonate, sodium bicarbonate, magnesium carbonate and the like were used. Now we began to understand why so many children responded to Buffered C (potassium bicarbonate, calcium carbonate, magnesium carbonate), and others needed a more specific buffer (in some children for example niacin was grossly depleted and they required niacin bicarbonate)," wrote Patricia Kane.

The simple household product used for baking, cleaning, bee stings and acid indigestion is so effective it sometimes prevent patients from having to be put on kidney machines. Or once on dialysis it makes the entire process a little easier.

Sodium bicarbonate is often used as an antacid taken orally to treat acid indigestion and heartburn. It may also be used in an oral form to treat chronic forms of metabolic acidosis such as chronic renal failure and renal tubular acidosis. Sodium bicarbonate may also be useful in urinary alkalinization for the treatment of aspirin overdose and uric acid renal stones.

In cases of respiratory acidosis, the infused bicarbonate ion drives the carbonic acid/bicarbonate buffer of plasma to the left and, thus, raises the pH. It is for this reason that sodium bicarbonate is used in medically-supervised cardiopulmonary resuscitation. Infusion of bicarbonate is indicated only when the blood pH is marked (< 7.1–7.0) low.

There are so many medical situations that sodium bicarbonate is helpful for. We will discuss the use of bicarbonate in the treatment of cancer, kidney disease, asthma, and diabetics but before we do we need to look at the fundamental reason sodium bicarbonate works so well and why having enough bicarbonate in the blood is important to our health.

2. The Four
Bicarbonate Sisters

The reduction of bicarbonates in the blood is the cause of aging and diseases, not the result of aging. As long as we can replenish bicarbonates in the blood, we don't have to age so fast. There are different ways we can increase bicarbonate concentrations with the use of sodium bicarbonate being the prominent way.

The bicarbonate transport system is a simple yet central part of our body's normal functioning. So it should come as no surprise that disruption of bicarbonate transport underlies many diseases.[1]

HCO_3^- is impermeable to biological membranes. Specialized plasma membrane bicarbonate transport proteins (bicarbonate transporter) are therefore required to facilitate HCO_3^- movement into and out of cells. Because HCO_3^- is a base, bicarbonate transporter-mediated influx induces cellular alkalization, while efflux causes acidification.

Physiologically the bicarbonate transport system serves to:

- regulate cellular pH,

- regulate whole body pH,

- regulate cell volume and fluid secretion,

- dispose of the body's major metabolic waste product (CO_2/HCO_3^-).

SODIUM, MAGNESIUM, POTASSIUM, AND CALCIUM

Sodium bicarbonate, and in fact all of the bicarbonates, are safe and easy to administer medicinals that have a profound effect on the body. There are four primary minerals in the body, sodium, magnesium, potassium and calcium and all four form bicarbonates. In the ocean, mammals use magnesium bicarbonate as the primary oxygen transporter since this mineral is the second most abundant in the ocean and sodium is carefully excluded from dominating physiology.

Sodium

Sodium bicarbonate is "only" 28 percent sodium, which means that for every 4 grams you ingest you get roughly 1 gram of sodium. Sodium is an essential nutrient required by the body for maintaining levels of fluids and for providing channels for nerve signaling. Some sodium is needed in your body to regulate fluids and blood pressure, and to keep muscles and nerves running smoothly.

Without appropriate amounts of sodium, your body may have a difficult time cooling down after intense exercise or activity. When the body is hot, you sweat. If you do not have enough sodium, your body may not sweat as much and you may then become overheated. This could then result in a stroke, exhaustion and dehydration.

Sodium is an energy carrier. It is also responsible for sending messages from the brain to muscles through the nervous system so that muscles move on command. When you want to move your arm or contract any muscle in your body, your brain sends a message to a sodium molecule that passes it to a potassium molecule and then back to a sodium molecule and so on, until it gets to its final destination and the muscle contracts. This is known as the sodium-potassium ion exchange. Therefore, without sodium, you would never be able to move any part of your body.

Excess sodium (such as that obtained from dietary sources) is excreted in the urine. Most of the sodium in the body (about 85 percent) is found in blood and lymph fluid. Sodium levels in the body are partly controlled by a hormone called aldosterone, which is made by the adrenal glands. Aldosterone levels determine whether the kidneys hold sodium in the body or pass it into the urine.

High Potassium-Low Sodium Diet

Dr. Max Gerson's daughter Charlotte Gerson said, "That sodium is never good, never in any form!" An essential component of Gerson's cancer therapy is the use of a low Na, high K diet. Dr. Freeman Cope wrote, "The high potassium, low sodium diet of the Gerson therapy has been observed experimentally to cure many cases of advanced cancer in man, but the reason was not clear. Recent studies from the laboratory of Ling indicate that high potassium, low sodium environments can partially return damaged cell proteins to their normal undamaged configuration. Therefore, the damage in other tissues, induced by toxins and breakdown products from cancer, is probably partly repaired by the Gerson therapy through this mechanism."

It is obvious from the Gerson diet that it is not all sodium they eliminate but high amounts of sodium that are frowned upon by Gerson. Sodium comes naturally from just about any kind of diet even that of raw foods. Charlotte got a little ahead of herself saying no sodium in any form because fruits and vegetables have sodium, which they use daily in copious quantities.

Importance of Sodium in One's Diet

Using sodium bicarbonate to brush ones teeth, as an emergency medicine or as a very inexpensive cancer treatment with the power to affect the body's alkalinity in days rather the weeks and months it takes to raise the body's pH with raw foods is good medicine. And it does not send up sodium or blood pressure levels because it is not the type of sodium (sodium chloride) that we have to be careful about. Refined table salt is harmful in high amounts and should be replaced with unrefined Real Salt, Celtic Salt or Himalayan salt.

Dr. David Brownstein, author of *Salt Your Way to Health* says, "My patients always give me quizzical looks when I tell them they need to increase their salt intake. You see, I have been checking salt levels on nearly every patient that has ever seen me. My experience has clearly shown that most patients do not consume enough salt. I know you are probably thinking that you read that last sentence incorrectly. We have been conditioned to think that we should eat less salt. The powers-that-be routinely release edicts stating that we need to eat less salt in order to be healthier and have less hypertension. However, that last statement is just not true. Eating less salt will not make us healthier and not lower the risk for hypertension. I have been writing about the importance of salt for well over fifteen years. Salt is the second major constituent in our body, next to water. We need adequate amounts of good salt in our diet to run hundreds of different biochemical pathways. Does salt cause blood pressure problems? The vast majority of people do not see any appreciable blood pressure lowering when they lower their salt intake. I quote many studies in my salt book which show the fallacy of lowering salt intake to lower blood pressure. There are a few individuals who are salt sensitive, but they are few and far between. In conventional medicine, salt consists of two ions, sodium and chloride. Refined salt is 99 percent sodium and chloride with toxic additives such as ferrocyanide and aluminum added to it. Unrefined salt is a better choice for salt because it contains essential minerals that are absent in refined salt products."

Bicarbonate Deficiencies

Bicarbonate deficiency is the most unrecognized medical condition on earth even though it is common. Problems revolving around acid pH levels (relative deficiency in bicarbonate ions) take a large toll on human physiology and the more acidic a person becomes, the larger the problem for their cells. Every biochemical reaction is pH sensitive, with enzymes being especially sensitive.

Dr. Lynda Frassetto talks about the most fundamental reason to use sodium bicarbonate and other mineral bicarbonates. "Insufficient amount of bicarbonates in our blood reduces our capabilities to manage (neutralize and dump) the acid our body produces. This is the cause of aging. The most important function of alkaline water is to increase bicarbonates in the blood because we lose bicarbonates as we age. As long as we can replenish bicarbonates in the blood, we don't have to age! Increase of bicarbonates in the bloodstream will prevent aging and the onset of adult degenerative diseases."

Even with healthy people a noticeable decline of bicarbonate begins at the age of 45. By age 90 we lose 18 percent of the bicarbonates in our blood. Bicarbonates are the alkaline buffers that neutralize acid, which results in the elimination of acidic waste in the body. Loss of bicarbonates hinders the blood from effectively managing the acid the body produces. This loss triggers the onset of acid-induced adult degenerative diseases such as acid reflux, kidney stones, diabetes, hypertension, osteoporosis, heart diseases, cancer, and gout.

The reduction of bicarbonates in the blood is the cause of aging and diseases, not the result of aging. As long as we can replenish bicarbonates in the blood, we don't have to age so fast. Since bicarbonates enter the bloodstream only when the stomach produces hydrochloric acid, it is important that we drink as much mineral rich alkaline water as possible, with the best waters high in bicarbonate and magnesium.

On an empty stomach, the stomach pH value may be high but the amount (volume) of hydrochloric acid in the stomach is small; therefore, drinking high pH (9.5 to 10) alkaline water will raise the stomach pH relatively high. This causes the stomach to produce more hydrochloric acid, allowing more bicarbonate to enter the bloodstream.

The change of pH value causes the stomach to produce hydrochloric acid that enters the stomach, and the bicarbonates enter the bloodstream.

When we say that we alkalize our body, we don't necessarily mean increasing our saliva pH or urine pH; it means increasing the bicarbonates in our blood. The blood pH does not change, but the ability of our blood to neutralize acid in the body increases quite dramatically.

SPARKLING WATER'S CHEMISTRY

Carbonated water contains dissolved CO_2 gas. Carbonated water is made by passing pressurized carbon dioxide through water. The main point to understand is the connection between drinking sparkling water, which has had CO_2 injected into it to make it fizzy, and drinking sodium bicarbonate in water, which turns to CO_2 in the stomach. People think drinking bicarbonate is a waste of time because it turns to CO_2 in the stomach but they could not be more mistaken.

Carbonation can occur naturally in spring water that picks up carbon dioxide stored in rocks, or it can be forced in by the manufacturer or by you at home with an inexpensive seltzer maker. Call it sparkling water, soda water, club soda or seltzer it's the same and those who avoid such drinks are missing a healthy and very delightful way to hydrate the body.

Scientific Findings

The Journal of Nutrition conducted a study of sparkling and still mineral water. The study participants were asked to drink one liter of either the sparkling or still each day for two months, followed by two months on the other water. It was found that drinking sparkling water[2] brought about significant reductions in the level of low density lipoprotein (LDL) cholesterol (generally regarded as a risk factor for heart disease), as well as a significant increase in levels of high density lipoprotein (HDL) cholesterol (generally taken to reduce heart disease risk). These and other biochemical changes induced by drinking sparkling water were estimated to reduce the women's risk of developing heart disease over the next decade by about one-third.[3]

During the study, the study participants underwent a number of tests including blood pressure checks and measurement of a variety of blood components including cholesterol. Interestingly, the Journal of Nutrition study found that the drinking of the sodium-rich mineral water did not lead to any increase in blood pressure. Sodium bicarbonate is not known to increase blood pressure despite the presence of sodium.

According to a study in the American Journal of Medicine the perfect water would have more than 48 milligrams of magnesium and 85 milligrams of calcium per liter, and fewer than 195 milligrams of sodium per liter. The perfect water would reverse that having twice as much calcium as magnesium.

Claims have been made that carbonated water erodes teeth and bones, leaches calcium and increases acidity in the stomach have not been borne out by experiment. In a healthy human, carbonation of water does not lead to ill health effects. In fact it is quite healthy and can be made even more so by adding more bicarbonate and magnesium to the mixture.

It is very simple to write off a good thing like bicarbonate when one does not understand the complexity of CO_2 and its relationship to bicarbonate. A lack of carbon dioxide (and thus oxygen) is a starting point for different disturbances in the body. If a carbon dioxide deficiency continues for a long time then it can be responsible for diseases, aging and cancer.

Dear Dr. Sircus,

"In the case of salt, in my studies on cancer I had interviewed Gerson patients that had experienced very good results on their therapy, and also read Max's book, etc. However, I noted that Charlotte only claims about 35 percent cure rates (recently) and I felt even though the cases were mostly extreme, the results could be a lot better. So I personally eliminated all salt from my already very clean, raw diet, and watched carefully. After a number of weeks my conclusion was that it caused a loss of energy and a possible loss of optimum water weight in the body, which I think could lead to other detrimental effects, as the right amount of water is needed for just about all functions. As soon as I added back the salt (Himalayan) the energy immediately returned, along with the water weight up to what seemed optimum. Endurance also improved back to normal."

Richard Sacks

We Need CO_2

Normal operation of the Krebs cycle produces CO_2 as a byproduct. When the Krebs cycle is interrupted, the absence of CO_2 creates deficiency in bicarbonate ions. We will spend several chapters discussing the relationships between bicarbonate, CO_2 and oxygen. It is basic that CO_2 respiration via carbonic acid through the lungs is a dominant acid control mechanism. Bicarbonate through the kidneys is the dominant alkali control mechanism for the blood.

A deficiency in CO_2 can adversely affect both acid and alkali balance systems. This dysfunction normally occurs when tissues tend towards anaerobic metabolism, resulting in elevated lactic acid-related acids and H+ ions. It also occurs when people breathe too quickly as all people with chronic illnesses and cancer do.

IMBLANCED pH CONDITIONS

Most modern diets give rise to unhealthy acidic pH conditions. An imbalanced pH will interrupt cellular activities and functions to extreme levels as pH drops further. Excessive acidic pH leads to cellular deterioration which eventually brings on serious health problems such as cancer, cardiovascular disease, diabetes, osteoporosis and heartburn. The fact that the biological life functions best in a non-acidic (alkaline) environment speaks miles about the usefulness of baking soda.

Health expert Sang Whang says, "The body's bicarbonate level remains fairly constant until the age of 45 and linearly decreases about 18 percent by the time one reaches 90 years of age. In general, adult degenerative diseases such as diabetes and high blood pressure start to appear at the age of 45 and up and gradually worsen approaching the age of 90 and up. It is this reduction of bicarbonates in the blood that affects blood flow and makes it difficult to manage the continuous outpour of acid, making it difficult to eliminate acid waste from the body and thereby developing many acid-induced degenerative diseases such as blood clots, acid reflux, heart disease, osteoporosis, gout, diabetes, high blood pressure, kidney disease, cancer, and strokes. Alzheimer's disease is nothing but a slow acidification of the brain. All these diseases are caused by systemic acidosis, which means insufficient bicarbonates in the blood."

When the body is bicarbonate-sufficient, it is more capable of resisting the toxicity of chemical insults and this is of course incredibly important with all the chemicals, heavy metals and the now-increasing radiation in our environment.

pH control is crucial for swimming pools. Pool alkalinity is the central part of pool water chemistry; therefore it is important that one tests it on regular basis. When you are correcting the total alkalinity level of a pool, it is recommended that we do so in small increments. Reason being, that it is much easier to adjust slightly when it gets a little high or a little low. Pool owners should not wait for their total alkalinity levels to get way off and then try to bring it back under control all at once.

Pool water care requires you to maintain a proper total alkalinity (TA) level at all times. If the TA is too low, Marbelite and plaster walls will become etched, metals corrode, the pool's walls and floor can stain, the water can turn green and ones eyes will burn. Doctors can learn from pool technicians how to diagnosis and treat the basic biochemistry of the body. They can send their patients home with these inexpensive pH strips so they can test the pH of their own fluids.

All of the cells in our body require the proper pH balance to function at an optimal level. If our body is acidic or too alkaline, chemical reactions including enzyme activity, cellular repair, and cellular reproduction are inhibited. Raymond Francis writes, "On the pH scale, 7 is neutral, 0 to 7 is acidic, and 7 to 14 is alkaline. The normal pH inside a cell is 7.4, which is slightly alkaline. Maintaining normal pH in the fluid inside the cell as well as the other body fluids is crucial for keeping the body systems functioning normally."

The blood is different. While most of the body can still operate outside of the optimum pH zone, blood cannot. Dr. Ian Shillington writes, "Your blood operates between 7.3 and 7.5 on the alkaline side of this pH scale. If it goes out of this range, you're dead!" And that's why they use sodium bicarbonate in emergency rooms and intensive care wards where life is threatened routinely. It will instantaneously bring someone back from the cliff's edge of death as the blood threatens to drop below a pH of 7.3.

Testing the pH Factor

By using pH test strips, you can determine your pH factor quickly and easily in the privacy of your own home. The first step with regards to pH medicine and using baking soda is to find out for sure if your body is acidic or not. If your body is acidic then follow the guidelines for restoring as near to 7.4 PH as you can. An acidic body can be implicated in much chronic ill health, including feeling tired. This is common in people who work and exercise too hard. An acid body is recognized as a factor in osteoarthritis and rheumatism. While the focus has traditionally been on acid foods, the problem is more due to the body being under capacity in its ability to buffer acidity. A healthy body should have no trouble tolerating acidic foods such as citrus and tomato.

To test the saliva, wait at least two hours after eating. Fill your mouth with saliva and then swallow it a couple of times before you put some saliva onto pH paper. The pH paper should turn blue, slightly alkaline at a healthy pH of 7.4. If it is not blue, compare the color with the chart that comes with the pH paper. If your saliva is acid (below pH of 7.0) wait two hours and repeat the test. The pH of a healthy person is in the 7.5 (dark blue) to 7.1 (blue) slightly alkaline range. The range from 6.5 (blue-green) is weakly acidic to 4.5 (light yellow) is strongly acidic. Most children are dark blue, a pH of 7.5.

If you are going to test urine: When urinary pH is continuously between 6.5 in the morning and 7.5 by evening, you are functioning in the healthy range. The blood plasma pH, under normal circumstances is slightly alkaline between 7.3 and 7.4. The urine tends to be a little lower with a healthy range of 6.8 to 7.0. Some believe the increased acidity of urine is reflective of the kidneys doing their job of excreting the excess acids in our body.

A highly acidic body can still be neutralized through the elimination of excessive acid and wastes from the body. This can be achieved by changing to a healthier diet. An alkaline-rich diet is the perfect diet program because an alkaline body can help reduce toxins and strengthen the immune system. In order to be completely healthy, we need to keep the chemical balance not only in our stomach but in our entire body system as well. Cleansing from the inside must be done to restore a healthy pH balance through the alkaline diet system for best long term results. We can assist and speed up this process with sodium bicarbonate though in the long run bicarbonate is not a substitute for a good alkaline diet.

Oral dosing of sodium bicarbonate is used to jump start the return of the body to a more healthy alkaline condition, followed by proper dietary intake of alkalinizing foods for maintenance. Sodium bicarbonate provides the body what it has been lacking in the Standard American Diet (SAD).

The recommendation is up to $1/8$ teaspoon per 8 ounce glass with a quarter slice of lemon (to balance the sodium with potassium) and no more than $1\frac{1}{2}$ to 2 teaspoons per 24-hour period.

pH Controls Key Cellular Pathways

In sport disciplines relying on speed endurance or strength endurance, anaerobic glycolysis provides the primary energy source for muscular contractions. The total capacity of the glycolytic pathway is limited by the progressive increase of acidity within the muscles, caused by the accumulation of hydrogen ions (Verbitsky et al., 1997). The increase in acidity ultimately inhibits energy transfer and the ability of the muscles to contract, forcing the athlete to decrease the intensity of exercise (Costill et al., 1984; Harrison and Thompson, 2005).[4]

In the life of a cell, the response to DNA damage determines whether the cell is fated to pause and repair itself, commit suicide, or grow uncontrollably, a route leading to cancer. A majority of genes in the mitochondrial, chaperone and proteasome pathways of nuclear DNA-encoded gene expression are decreased with decreased brain pH.

Dr. Robert O. Young, Director of Research at the pH Miracle Living Center suggests, "All genetic changes within any cell are always the result of an acidic change in the environment surrounding that cell. These cellular changes are generally caused by acidic contributing factors such as primary or secondary acidic smoke from cigarettes or living and/or working in acidic polluted environments. The best way to protect any cell from acidic genetic change that can lead to a cancerous condition is to maintain the delicate alkaline pH of the fluids surrounding that cell with an alkaline lifestyle and diet."

Symptoms of Acid Conditions

Acidic change in the body shows up in many different ways. The following conditions—Beginning Symptoms, Intermediate Symptoms, and Advanced Symptons—are common to bodies that are overly acidic:

Beginning Symptoms

- Acne
- Agitation
- Bloating
- Chemical sensitivities to odor, gas heat
- Cold hands and feet
- Constipation
- Diarrhea
- Dizziness
- Excess head mucous (stuffiness)
- Food allergies
- Hard to get up in morning
- Heartburn
- Hot urine
- Hyperactivity
- Irregular heartbeat
- Joint pains that travel
- Lack of sex drive
- Low energy
- Metallic taste in mouth
- Mild headaches
- Muscular pain
- Panic attacks
- Pre-menstrual and menstrual cramping
- Pre-menstrual anxiety and depression
- Rapid heartbeat
- Rapid panting breath
- Strong smelling urine
- White coated tongue

Intermediate Symptoms

- Asthma
- Bacterial infections (staph, strep)
- Bronchitis
- Cold sores (Herpes I & II)
- Colitis
- Cystitis
- Depression

- Disturbance in smell, taste, vision, hearing
- Ear aches
- Endometriosis
- Excessive falling hair
- Fungal infections (Candia albicans, athlete's foot, vaginal)
- Gastritis
- Hay fever
- Hives
- Impotence
- Insomnia
- Loss of concentration
- Loss of memory
- Migraine headaches
- Numbness and tingling
- Psoriasis
- Sinusitis
- Stuttering
- Swelling
- Urethritis
- Urinary infection
- Viral infections (colds, flu)

Advanced Symptoms

- All other forms of cancer
- Crohn's disease
- Hodgkin's Disease
- Learning disabled
- Leukemia
- Multiple Sclerosis
- Myasthenia gravis
- Rheumatoid arthritis
- Sarcoidosis
- Schizophrenia
- Scleroderma
- Systemic Lupus Erythematosis
- Tuberculosis

Source: *Alkalize or Die,* Dr. Theodore A. Baroody,1991.

Understanding that your body is trying to tell you something through the symptoms it presents is an important step in identifying an underlying problem. Treating only the symptoms without alleviating the cause will not make the problem go away. By observing these specific conditions as detailed above, you can see whether or not the problem stems from a pH imbalance. Once you have identified the problem, as you will see in the next chapter, you have a safe treatment available in the form of sodium bicarbonate.

3. Basic Uses of Sodium Bicarbonate

Sodium bicarbonate is often found in household cleaners and laundry detergents because of its ability to lift dirt and grime, and its efficacy in eliminating unpleasant odors. It is no surprise that this magic powder is the most effective and economical way to clean oil-stained clothes.

Baking soda has literally hundreds of uses. A paste from baking soda can be very effective when used in cleaning and scrubbing. It removes coffee stains, marker, and crayon. It can be used to clean out grease. A solution in warm water will remove the tarnish from silver when the silver is in contact with a piece of aluminum foil. It even acts as a fire-suppression agent in some dry powder fire extinguishers.

As an absorbent for moisture and odors, an open box can be left in a refrigerator for this purpose. In toothpaste, baking soda helps to gently remove stains, whiten teeth, it freshens the breath, and dissolve plaque. In fact, sodium bicarbonate, used in more and more toothpastes and in newer teeth-cleaning devices, is the very best agent for the maintenance of oral health because it changes pH, radically disrupting the constantly rising tide of bacteria and fungi that threaten the health status of the entire body. With ample brushing, sodium bicarbonate has the power to break through pathogen films, called biofilms,[1] that sticky stuff that turns into hard tarter that your dentist has to struggle to remove while you grin and bear it.

Sodium bicarbonate is even effective as cerumenolytic ear drops.[2] It can also be used as a mouth rinse which can then be swallowed. Canker sores (aphthous ulcers) are tiny ulcerations that occur in the oral cavity on or near the tongue and on the inner mucous membrane of the lip. They can be very painful to the point of interfering with speech and eating. They also tend to heal slowly. The source of the problem is usually an acid condition in the body caused by food or chemical allergies. Sodium bicarbonate is effective for canker sores and ulcers.

With water, it cleans the impurities on contact lenses. Rinse completely before wearing contacts to avoid stinging of the salt in baking soda. Baking soda and boiling water unclogs drains. One cup of baking soda maintains a healthy septic tank. It controls pH and keeps a good environment for the bacteria. If made into a paste salve, it relieves burning from bug stings, poison ivy, nettles, and sunburn. It kills fleas and drives away ants. If it is applied to a pet's fur, it must be washed/rinsed off to prevent skin problems. A small amount can be added to a beef stew to make tough meat tenderize faster. It is used as a fabric softener in laundry.

The native chemical and physical properties of sodium bicarbonate account for its wide range of applications, including cleaning, deodorizing, buffering, and fire extinguishing. Sodium bicarbonate neutralizes odors chemically, rather than masking them. Consequently, it is used in bath salts and deodorant body powders. Sodium bicarbonate tends to maintain a pH of 8.1 (7 is neutral) even when acids, which lower pH, or bases, which raise pH, are added to the solution. It is commonly used to increase the pH and total alkalinity of the water for pools and spas.

Sodium bicarbonate, the monosodium salt of carbonic acid, is used as a gastric and systemic antacid and to alkalize urine; also used, in solution, for washing the nose, mouth, and vagina, as a cleansing enema, and as a dressing for minor burns.

Many Common Usages

For Your Food

- baking
- produce wash
- sports drink

Cleaning

- drain cleaner
- absorbs odors in the fridge
- clean toilets
- scouring sinks/tubs/counters
- clean pots/pans
- remove hard water stains
- deodorize garbage disposal
- freshen carpets
- deodorize microwave
- clean coffeemaker
- polish silver tea set
- clean flat top stove
- cut grease on dishes
- mop floors

Laundry

- laundry booster
- cloth diapers
- remove armpit stains
- freshen stuffed animals

For Kids

- model volcanoes
- water color paints
- bath fizzies
- play clay
- magic beans
- cork races

Health & Beauty

- relieve heartburn
- detox bath
- itch relief
- bee/wasp stings
- toothpaste
- deodorant
- facial exfoliant
- no-shampoo hair care
- remove dirt/stains from hands/feet
- relieve leg cramps
- gargle during a cold
- fever reducer
- clean retainers/dentures
- clean brushes/combs
- clean glasses
- teeth whitener
- breath freshener

Around the House

- absorb odors in shoes
- deodorize litterbox
- eliminate skunk odor
- pesticide
- rabbit deterrent in the garden
- slug killer
- clean grills
- remove oil and grease stains
- car cleaner
- deodorize RV water tank
- restore paintbrushes
- clean white boards
- remove crayon/marker from walls
- flower food
- put out small kitchen fires
- deodorize trash can/diaper pail

Natural Emergency and Intensive Care Medicines

Some of the secrets of emergency room and intensive care medicine hold the key to the safe practice of medicine. Magnesium salts, sodium bicarbonate, iodine, selenium and vitamin C are concentrated nutritional medicinals that have been used in the direst of medical circumstances either by intramuscular (IM) injection or intravenous feed. But are these substances really medicines?

One reader wrote:

Dr. Sircus, you list the following: "Magnesium chloride, sodium bicarbonate (baking soda), selenium, sulfur, iodine, glutathione and vitamin C in your most recent post and then claim, "Every one of the above medicines can be used to great advantage." Since when are the minerals selenium, sulfur, iodine classified as "medicines"—or glutathione, which is made naturally in the human body? People think of medicines as the poisons produced by the pharmaceutical professions and minerals, vitamins, and other supplements as natural substances provided by God. Could you please explain your use of the word "medicines" in the same context with vitamins and minerals?

The very reason I named my medical approach "Natural Allopathic Medicine" answers this question. Very few doctors will get on the horn and tell everyone how wonderful magnesium salts are in the emergency room because it is a substance taken directly from the sea. Legally if you inject magnesium salts or administer them intravenously, they are considered a medicine and you need a medical license to perform such procedures. The same of course can be said for bicarbonate. Magnesium and bicarbonates are used as medicines because they are medicines, though we could call them medicinals. Magnesium chloride and different forms of bicarbonate are actually found in seawater, which itself makes a great emergency room medicine.

During World War II, Navy doctors would use seawater for blood transfusions when blood supplies ran out, and many lives were saved.

We create medicines when we concentrate things in nature. Pharmaceutical companies concentrate synthetic substances, which does not work out very well for patients in the end. Natural Allopathic Medicine concentrates elements from nature that are proven by scientists to offer powerful healing without toxic side effects. One cannot say that about any pharmaceutical, for even aspirin kills 15,000 a year in the United States alone.

Deep within the heart of western medicine is a wisdom and power that is deliberately stymied by medical authorities and the pharmaceutical companies that stand behind them. Inside the emergency room and intensive care wards, where many believe some of the most accurate medicine is practiced, are common but extraordinarily safe and effective substances that save lives every day. Interesting no one has thought to harness these medical super weapons against chronic disease or cancer.

Sodium bicarbonate is a prime example of this type of medicine. It is used every day in every good hospital of the world because it is safe, effective, and does a medical job no other substance can do. In the emergency room medicines have to be safe while delivering an instant lifesaving burst of healing power. Obviously if they are safe and strong enough for emergency situations they are going to help us with chronic diseases and acute ones as well.

Sodium bicarbonate, potassium chloride, and calcium chloride are used to maintain pH and electrolytes within normal values in intensive care units.

When the nervous system is injured, the brain produces self-protective molecules in an attempt to halt damage. Following injury, the death of nerve cells occurs over a prolonged period of many hours or days, which provides a "window" for therapeutic intervention.

Research suggests that administering sodium bicarbonate in intravenous (IV) form can significantly improve pH and PCO_2 in children with life-threatening asthma. Respiratory distress and level of consciousness both improved after the administration of sodium bicarbonate.[3]

Sodium Bicarbonate Injection: USP is administered by the intravenous route. In cardiac arrest, a rapid intravenous dose of one to two 50 mL vials (44.6 to 100 mEq) may be given initially and continued at a rate of 50 mL (44.6 to 50 mEq) every 5 to 10 minutes if necessary (as indicated by arterial pH and blood gas monitoring) to reverse the acidosis. Caution should be observed in emergencies where very rapid infusion of large quantities of bicarbonate is indicated. Bicarbonate solutions are hypertonic and may produce an undesirable rise in plasma sodium concentration in the process of correcting the metabolic acidosis. In cardiac arrest, however, the risks from acidosis exceed those of hypernatremia. Two minutes after intubation, premature ventricular contractions, ventricular fibrillation, bradycardia, and finally cardiac arrest were recognized. An increase of serum potassium from 3.19 to 8.64 mmol/L was observed in arterial blood. The patient was immediately resuscitated with chest compressions, intravenous adrenaline, atropine, lidocaine, and sodium bicarbonate.[4]

Magnesium chloride can be administered orally, transdermally, or intravenously. Intramuscular injection is also possible but can be painful. Oral administration of a daily dose of more than 50 mmol can cause vomiting and diarrhea. In anesthesia and intensive care, the preferred administration route is IV.

When magnesium is used to correct a magnesium deficit, the objective is to restore normal serum concentrations, in which case a slow infusion of up to 10 gm/day is appropriate. When replacing magnesium via the IV route, approximately half of the dose is retained by the body while the remainder is excreted in the urine. The low retention rate is due to the slow uptake of magnesium by cells and decreased magnesium reabsorption by the kidneys in response to the delivery of a large concentration of magnesium.[5]

In my essay *Avoiding Heart Disease & Strokes* I explain more of the necessity for magnesium in heart disease and how doctors are neglecting to embrace this important mineral resulting in a significant lack of success over the past decade in treating heart failure. Magnesium should be taken for all conditions of the heart except for when the blood pressure is too low or the threat of kidney failure is present. Since there is no drug that can substitute for magnesium it is indicated for the majority of heart patients particularly in its chloride form and in its magnesium bicarbonate form. This is the definitive medicine for both the prevention and treatment of heart disease.

Dr. Boris Veysman, specialist in emergency medicine at the Robert Wood Johnson University Hospital in New Jersey, describes one emergency room experience: "The emergency department is always noisy, but today the triage nurse is yelling 'not breathing,' as she runs toward us pushing a wheelchair. A pale, thin woman is slumped over and looking gray. Without concrete proof of a 'Do Not Resuscitate' order, there's no hesitation. Click, klang, and the patient has a tube down her throat within seconds. I do the chest compressions. On the monitor, she is flat-lining—no heartbeat. I synchronize my words with the compressions and call out for an external pacemaker. Pumping . . . thinking: Cardiac standstill . . . after walking in . . . with cancer . . . on chemo. This resuscitation isn't by the book.' Get two amps of bicarbonate,' I say to the intern. The jugular line takes seconds, and I flush it with sodium bicarbonate. This probably will correct the blood's extreme acidity, which I suspect is driving up the potassium. The external pacemaker finally arrives. Potent electric shocks at 80 beats per minute begin to stimulate her heart. The vitals stabilize.[6]

Sodium bicarbonate is an emergency room intensive care medicine that can be used in cancer treatment as well as in fighting the symptoms of the flu. It is not though a permanent substitute for dietary corrections that lead to a healthy alkaline existence but it can be used quite effectively to change the terrain of tissues and cells quickly. Caution should be observed in emergencies where very rapid infusion of large quantities of bicarbonate is indicated. Bicarbonate solutions are hypertonic and may produce an undesirable rise in plasma sodium concentration in the process of correcting the metabolic acidosis. In cardiac arrest, however, the risks from acidosis exceed those of hypernatremia.

Sodium bicarbonate injection is indicated in the treatment of metabolic acidosis, which may occur in severe renal disease, uncontrolled diabetes, and circulatory insufficiency due to shock or severe dehydration, extracorporeal circulation of blood, cardiac arrest, and severe primary lactic acidosis. Sodium bicarbonate is further indicated in the treatment of drug intoxications, including barbiturates. Sodium bicarbonate is effective in treating poisonings from or overdoses of many chemicals and pharmaceutical drugs by negating the cardiotoxic and neurotoxic effects.[7]

Bicarbonate is used routinely in:

- Severe diabetic ketoacidosis[8]
- Cardiopulmonary resuscitation[9]
- Pregnancy[10]
- Hemodialysis[11]
- Peritoneal dialysis[12]
- Pharmacological toxicosis[13]
- Hepatopathy[14]
- Vascular surgery operations[15]

The pH of solid tumors is acidic due to increased fermentative metabolism and poor perfusion. It has been hypothesized that acid pH promotes local invasive growth and metastasis. The hypothesis that acid mediates invasion proposes that H^+ diffuses from the proximal tumor microenvironment into adjacent normal tissues where it causes tissue remodeling that permits local invasion.

Bicarbonate ions create the conditions for increased glucose transport across cell plasma membranes. It also helps magnesium get into the mitochondria. Bicarbonate ions also create the alkaline conditions for maintaining the enzyme activity of pancreatic secretions in the intestines thus it should be of benefit in the treatment of pancreatitis. Bicarbonate ions neutralize the acid conditions required for chronic inflammatory reactions. Bicarbonate ions modify the acid conditions in osteoclast cells in bone and modify the acid conditions in Synovial Type A cells in joints, thus it should be of benefit in the treatment of osteoporosis, osteoarthritis, and even bone cancer.

4. The Pancreas, Diabetes, and Bicarbonate

Understanding of sodium bicarbonate begins with a trip to the pancreas, which is the organ most responsible for producing the bicarbonate our bodies need. Naturopath Parhatsathid Napatalung from Thailand writes, "The pancreas is harmed if the body is metabolically acid as it tries to maintain bicarbonates. Without sufficient bicarbonates, the pancreas is slowly destroyed, insulin becomes a problem and hence diabetes becomes an issue. Without sufficient bicarbonate buffer, the effect of disease is far reaching as the body becomes acid." Type 1 diabetes results from an immune-mediated destruction of pancreatic [beta]-cells, but the initiating causes are unknown to western science but that does not mean the causes have to remain unknown to you.

Drinking tap water or any acid demineralized water is going to take one to their grave a lot faster than drinking high alkaline high pH highly mineralized water will. Tap water pH 6.2–6.9 is associated with a *fourfold higher risk of type 1 diabetes* compared with pH ≥7.7. Drinking the wrong type of water, water lacking in bicarbonates and magnesium will contribute to the onset of many diseases. When we look at the fact that the quality of drinking water influences the risk of type 1 diabetes we are looking simultaneously down at heart disease, strokes and cancer because the chances of contracting these diseases increases for diabetic patients.

Increased oxidative stress, *which correlates almost exponentially with pH changes into the acidic,* is especially dangerous to the mitochondria, which suffer the greatest under oxidative duress. Bicarbonate acts to stimulate the ATPase by acting directly on the mitochondria[1] so bicarbonate deficiencies (acid conditions) affect mitochondrial activity.

Dr. Burt Berkson, licensed by the FDA to do research into intravenous Alpha Lipoic Acid, talking about free radical damage says "When the damage occurs in the pancreas, it may lead to diabetes. When it takes place in the heart, coronary heart disease may result." Free radicals are like the dust that collects under the rug. Over the years the dust collects and then things can get so filthy that bacteria collect as well as mold and mildew.

On August 1, 2006, the American Chemical Society published research that showed conclusively that Methyl mercury induces pancreatic cell apoptosis and dysfunction. Organic mercury creates a considerable amount of oxidative stress and free radical damage.

Logically there are just certain areas that are worse than others and in some places things just get out of control as literally a fire burns down cellular houses and certainly healthy cellular function. At such places in the body we might expect to see a cancer develop, a rapidly growing colony of cells that is just feeding on the filth and on cellular weakness, tissues severely disturbed with deficiencies of vital minerals an antioxidants.

PANCREAS

The pancreas is a long, narrow gland which stretches from the spleen to about the middle of the duodenum. It has three main functions. Firstly, it is to provide digestive juices, which contain pancreatic enzymes in an alkaline solution to provide the right conditions for the digestive process to be completed in the small intestines.

Secondly, the pancreas produces insulin, the hormone which controls blood sugar by the metabolism of sugar and other carbohydrates. Thirdly, it produces bicarbonate to neutralize acids coming from the stomach to provide the right environment for the pancreatic enzymes to be effective.

Allergies generally start with the body's inability to produce a certain enzyme, or to produce enough enzymes for the digestive process to work effectively. In conjunction with this is an inability to produce enough bicarbonate essential for the pancreatic enzymes to function properly. When this happens undigested proteins penetrate the bloodstream inducing more allergic reactions. Inflammation in such a scenario is systemic, but can focus on the pancreas forcing decreases in the production of bicarbonate, insulin and necessary enzymes.[2]

Importance of Bicarbonate

The bicarbonate ion acts as a buffer to maintain the normal levels of acidity (pH) in blood and other fluids in the body. Body alkalinity is affected by foods or medications that we ingest and the function of the kidneys and lungs. The normal serum range for bicarbonate is 22 to 30 mmol/L.

Disruptions in normal bicarbonate levels may be due to diseases that interfere with respiratory function, kidney diseases, metabolic conditions and a failing pancreas. The pancreas, an organ largely responsible for pH control,[3] is one of the first organs affected when general pH shifts to the acidic. "Monitoring of blood-sugar levels, insulin production, acid-base balance, and pancreatic bicarbonate and enzyme production before and after test exposures to potentially allergic substances reveals that the *pancreas is the first organ to develop inhibited function from varied stresses*,[4] writes Dr. William Philpott and Dr. Dwight K. Kalita in their book *Brain Allergies*.

Dr. Robert Young, states, "Excess acidity is a condition that weakens all body systems. The pancreas is one of our body's organs charged with the awesome responsibility to 'alkalinize' us. Can you start to see how our serious acidosis has overwhelmed our pancreas' ability to operate effectively, which then results in a state called 'diabetes?'

Vulnerable Pancreas

Pancreatic secretion of bicarbonate decreases in severe malnutrition in spite of increased flow rate of pancreatic secretion.[5] When one of many possible biological stresses weigh down the pancreas it will, as any other organ will, begin to function improperly. When this happens the first thing we will see is a reduction in pancreatic bicarbonate production.

Once there is an inhibition of pancreatic function and pancreatic bicarbonate flow there naturally follows a chain reaction of inflammatory reactions throughout the body. The reactions would include the brain as acidic conditions begin to generally prevail. Decreasing bicarbonate flow would boomerang on the pancreas, which itself needs proper alkaline conditions to provide the full amount of bicarbonate necessary for the body.

A highly acidic pH level puts the pancreas, liver, and all the body's organs at risk. Because of the important role played by the liver in removing acid waste from the body, liver function is also particularly at risk when acids accumulate. When acidity prevents the liver and pancreas from regulating blood sugar, the risk of diabetes and thus cancer will increase.

DIABETES

There are many causes of diabetes. Heavy metals, toxic chemicals, and radiation contamination will affect, weaken, and destroy pancreatic tissues. When the body is bicarbonate sufficient it is more capable of resisting the toxicity of chemical insults. That is why the army suggests its use to protect the kidneys from radiological contamination.[6] Much the same can be said for magnesium levels. Magnesium, bicarbonate, and iodine all protect us from the constant assault of noxious chemicals and radiation exposure we are subjected to everyday in our water, food, and air.

Diabetes is a fundamental disease that affects the entire colony of cells in a person because it has to do with energy metabolism and the vastly important hormone insulin and its receptor sites. Diabetes is actually an extremely serious warning to civilization; it is an announcement that the rising tide of radiation, mercury, other deadly chemicals and pharmaceutical drugs are poisoning humanity. We even have to look at how antibiotics are leading to diabetes as well as a host of other problems for the human body. These toxic insults are slamming head on to nutritional deficiencies in the body and the results are telling though still being ignored by the orthodox medical establishment, which has its heart dead set on adding not subtracting to these insult.

Dr. Lisa Landymore-Lim in her book *Poisonous Prescriptions* explains how many drugs used by the unsuspecting public today, are involved in the onset of impaired glucose control and diabetes. She explains using the example of the drugs streptozocin and alloxan, which are both used in research to make lab rats diabetic. Vacor is a rat poison known to cause insulin dependent diabetes in humans. Allopathic medicine will eventually have to face up to the fact that many drugs, including most surprisingly, the antibiotics including penicillin, as well as an entire host of others, causes changes in the beta cells affecting both insulin and bicarbonate production.

Treatment of Diabetes with Bicarbonate

Sodium bicarbonate dramatically slows the progress of chronic kidney disease but few have followed the conclusion that it would also be a front line defense against diabetes. From prevention to treatment and to part of a cure, common baking soda is an essential tool in working with diabetic and metabolic syndromes.

Pancreatic secretion of bicarbonate decreases in severe malnutrition and it is known that most obese people are malnourished. The famous junk food diet that leads to diabetes is a diet guaranteed to create malnutrition and thus decreased bicarbonate flow as well as severe magnesium deficiencies, which itself is a major cause of diabetes. The more acidic the foods the more bicarbonate is needed; so the pancreas gets further and further behind as the demand increases for alkaline buffers.

Sodium bicarbonate injections are already indicated in the treatment of metabolic acidosis, which may occur in severe renal disease, uncontrolled diabetes, circulatory insufficiency due to shock or severe dehydration, extracorporeal circulation of blood, cardiac arrest, and severe primary lactic acidosis. But sodium bicarbonate can be used safely at home orally and transdermally (and should always be used with magnesium for greatest effect) during all stages of diabetes. In addition, sodium bicarbonate baths may be used in treating the diabetic foot (see page 82).

Improper pH balance puts diabetics at greater risk for complications such as kidney failure, gangrene, and blindness. A diabetic suffers from an excess of glucose in the bloodstream, glucose that cannot be delivered properly to the body's cells due to lack of insulin. As the liver absorbs more and more of the excess glucose, its ability to remove toxins from the body becomes impaired.

5. Sodium Bicarbonate and Kidney Disease

The kidneys are usually the first organs to show chemical damage upon uranium exposure. Old military manuals suggest doses or infusions of sodium bicarbonate to help alkalinize the urine if this happens. This makes the uranyl ion less kidney-toxic and promotes excretion of the nontoxic uranium-carbonate complex. The oral administration of sodium bicarbonate diminishes the severity of the changes produced by uranium in the kidneys.[1]

The exocrine section of the pancreas has been greatly ignored in the treatment of diabetes even though its impairment is a well-documented condition. It is primarily responsible for the production of enzymes and bicarbonate necessary for normal digestion of food. Bicarbonate is so important for protecting the kidneys that even the kidneys get into the act of producing bicarbonate and now we know the common denominator between diabetes and kidney disease. When the body is hit with reductions in bicarbonate output by these two organs, acid conditions build and then entire body physiology begins to go south.

Acid-Base Balance

The kidneys alone produce about two hundred and fifty grams (about half a pound) of bicarbonate per day in an attempt to neutralize acid in the body. The kidneys monitor and control the acidity or "acid-base" (pH) balance of the blood. If the blood is too acidic, the kidney makes bicarbonate to restore the bloods pH balance. If the blood is too alkaline, then the kidney excretes bicarbonate into the urine to restore the balance. Acid-base balance is the net result of two processes, first, the removal of bicarbonate subsequent to hydrogen ion production from the metabolism of dietary constituents; second, the synthesis of "new" bicarbonate by the kidney.[2]

Substituting a sodium bicarbonate solution for saline infusion prior to administration of radiocontrast material seems to reduce the incidence of nephropathy.[3]
—Dr. Thomas P. Kennedy, American Medical Association

It is considered that normal adults eating ordinary Western diets have chronic, low-grade acidosis which increases with age. This excess acid, or acidosis, is considered to contribute to many diseases and to contribute to the aging process. Acidosis occurs often when the body cannot produce enough bicarbonate ions (or other alkaline compounds) to neutralize the acids in the body formed from metabolism and drinking highly acid drinks like Coke, Pepsi, and all the rest of them. High protein diets are also a problem in this regard and in the long run give the kidneys a run for their money.

Acid-buffering by means of base supplementation is one of the major roles of dialysis. Bicarbonate concentration in the dialysate (solution containing water and chemicals (electrolytes) that passes through the artificial kidney to remove excess fluids and wastes from the blood, also called "bath.") should be personalized in order to reach a midweek pre-dialysis serum bicarbonate concentration of 22 mmol/l.[4] Use of sodium bicarbonate in dialysate has been shown in studies to better control some metabolic aspects and to improve both treatment tolerance and patients' life quality. Bicarbonate dialysis, unlike acetate-free biofiltration, triggers mediators of inflammation and apoptosis.[5]

One of the main reasons we become acidic is from over-consumption of protein. Research suggests eating meat and dairy products may increase the risk of prostate cancer.[6] We would find the same for breast and other cancers as well. Conversely mineral deficiencies are another reason and when you combine high protein intake with decreasing intake of minerals you have a medical disaster in the making through lowering of pH into highly acidic conditions. When protein breaks down in our bodies they break into strong acids.

Unless a treatment actually removes acid toxins from the body and increases oxygen, water, and nutrients most medical interventions come to naught. These acids must be excreted by the kidneys because they contain sulfur, phosphorus or nitrogen which cannot break down into water and carbon dioxide to be eliminated as the weak acids are. In their passage through the kidneys these strong acids must take a basic mineral with them because in this way they are converted into their neutral salts and don't burn the kidneys on their way out. This would happen if these acids were excreted in their free acid form.

Importance of Bicarbonates

Bicarbonate ions neutralize the acid conditions required for chronic inflammatory reactions. Hence, sodium bicarbonate is of benefit in the treatment of a range of chronic inflammatory and autoimmune diseases. Sodium bicarbonate is a scientific medicine with known effects. When a treatment can be looked at in a scientific light it can be more easily accepted. Sodium bicarbonate is effective in treating poisonings or overdoses from many chemicals and pharmaceutical drugs by also negating the cardiotoxic and neurotoxic effects.[7] It is the main reason it is used by orthodox oncology—to mitigate the highly toxic effects of chemotherapy.

Sodium bicarbonate possesses the property of absorbing heavy metals, dioxins and furans. Comparison of cancer tissue with healthy tissue from the same person shows that the cancer tissue has a much higher concentration of toxic chemicals, pesticides, and other toxic materials. Sodium bicarbonate injection is indicated in the treatment of metabolic acidosis which may occur in severe renal disease, uncontrolled diabetes, and circulatory insufficiency due to shock or severe dehydration, extracorporeal circulation of blood, cardiac arrest, and severe primary lactic acidosis. The acid/alkaline balance is one of the most overlooked aspects of health, though many have written much about it. In general, the American public is heavily acidic, excepting vegetarians, and even their bodies have to face increasing levels of toxic exposure.

These bicarbonates are the alkaline buffers that neutralize excess acids in the blood; they dissolve solid acid wastes into liquid form. As they neutralize the solid acidic wastes, extra carbon dioxide is released, which is discharged through the lungs. As our body gets old, these alkaline buffers get low; this phenomenon is called acidosis. This is a natural occurrence as our body accumulates more acidic waste products. There is, therefore, a relationship between the aging process and the accumulation of acids.

It is not a good idea to forget the acid side of the equation and push the body too high into the alkaline state for too long. There are limits to everything and one should not ignore the two week maximum dosage that is on the box of Arm & Hammer's sodium bicarbonate. One patient on a do or die alkaline program (not using sodium bicarbonate) wrote, "Now after 3 weeks of having morning urine pH higher then 8, I have many discomforts in the whole organism including headache, pain in muscular and joints, and problem with digestive system." The bicarbonate treatment goes for a maximum of two weeks and does not seek to maintain such high pH values for long periods of time, though after a week to ten days off of intensive bicarbonate therapy one can do the protocol again.

A stable bicarbonate dialysis solution for peritoneal dialysis contains bicarbonate, calcium, and magnesium. This bicarbonate-based solution is stable over long periods.[8]

Scientific Findings

Researchers from Department of Medicine and General Clinical Research Center, University of California[9] have found, "Renal insufficiency induces metabolic acidosis by reducing conservation of filtered bicarbonate and excretion of acid. With advancing age, the severity of diet-dependent acidosis increases independently of diet.[10] That occurs because kidney function ordinarily declines substantially with age, resulting in a condition similar to that of chronic renal insufficiency."[11]

Research by British scientists at the Royal London Hospital has shown that sodium bicarbonate can dramatically slow the progress of chronic kidney disease. The *Journal of the American Society of Nephrology* clearly understands the efficacy of bicarbonate in treating kidney disease and so do many practicing nephrologists.

Dr. S. K. Hariachar, a nephrologist who oversees the Renal Hypertension Unit in Tampa, Florida stated, upon seeing the research on bicarbonate and kidney disease, "I am glad to see confirmation of what we have known for so long. I have been treating my patients with bicarbonate for many years in attempts to delay the need for dialysis, and now we finally have a legitimate study to back us up. We have the added information that some people already on dialysis can reverse their condition with the use of sodium bicarbonate."

John, a dialysis technician at the same center as Dr. Hariachar, who used to be on dialysis himself for two years as a result of kidney failure, had his kidneys miraculously start functioning to the point where dialysis was no longer needed. He states that he was prescribed oral doses of sodium bicarbonate throughout his treatment and still takes it daily to prevent recurrences of kidney failure. Dr. Hariachar maintains, though, that not everyone will be helped by taking bicarbonate. He says that those patients who have difficulty excreting acids, even with dialysis using a bicarbonate dialysate bath, that, "oral bicarbonate makes all the difference."

Sodium bicarbonate lessens the development of polycystic kidney disease in rats. Chronic administration of sodium bicarbonate to rats inhibited cystic enlargement and prevented the subsequent development of interstitial inflammation, chronic fibrosis, and uremia.[12]

6. *Using Sodium Bicarbonate as a Therapeutic Agent*

The only problem with sodium bicarbonate is that Arm & Hammer baking soda can replace many more expensive medicines and this does not make pharmaceutical executives happy at all. Sodium bicarbonate has been valued as a therapeutic agent for colds and influenza, stomach ailments, radiation, chemical and heavy metal toxicity, and oral hygiene, as well as its other uses.

The controversy over sodium bicarbonate and its role as a medical treatment might be relatively new, but baking soda has a long history of use. *The Eloquent Peasant*, an Egyptian story that dates to around 2000 BC, refers to a peddler selling natron, a natural blend of sodium bicarbonate, chloride, and sodium carbonate that was used in mummification—just one of hundreds of ways baking soda has been utilized. Baking soda's first widespread use, however, was probably as a leavening agent for bread and other baked goods. It has been used commercially since 1775, although the now-famous Arm & Hammer brand wasn't introduced until 1867.

The wide use of sodium bicarbonate as a home remedy extends back to the days when baking soda, iodine, and cannabinoid medicine lined the shelves of pharmacies. Sodium bicarbonate-medicated baths have been one of the first lines of treatment for psoriasis, even with sophisticated immuno-suppressive treatments available.

The effectiveness of sodium bicarbonate baths in psoriasis treatment was demonstrated when thirty-one patients with mild-moderate psoriasis were studied. Of these patients, a majority who used the baking soda remedy reported significant improvements in symptoms. These baths alleviated enough of the suffering of psoriasis that the subjects continued to include sodium bicarbonate in their treatment after the study had ended.[1]

I have had Morgellons for over 6 years—very nasty—and I know you are aware of our plight. I am now ready to start your transdermal magnesium therapy treatments but first I have to tell you something. I would like you to know that *bicarbonate baths really help me.* But, I use it with about 3 lbs of sea salt per bath, because when I did 5 lbs of bicarbonate I put myself into an alkaline state. The high salt content somehow opened up my skin to take in the bicarbonate, and it came out of my skin for a few weeks!

C D

COLDS AND INFLUENZA

In a 1926 booklet,[2] published by the Arm & Hammer Soda Company. On page 12 the company says, "The proven value of Arm & Hammer Bicarbonate of Soda as a therapeutic agent was championed by a prominent physician named Dr. Volney S. Cheney, in a letter to the Church & Dwight Company:

In 1918 and 1919 while fighting the 'Flu' with the U.S. Public Health Service it was brought to my attention that rarely anyone who had been thoroughly alkalinized with bicarbonate of soda contracted the disease, and those who did contract it, if alkalinized early, would invariably have mild attacks. I have since that time treated all cases of 'Cold,' 'Influenza' and 'LaGripe' by first giving generous doses of Bicarbonate of Soda, and in many, many instances within 36 hours the symptoms would have entirely abated. Further, within my own household, before Woman's Clubs and Parent-Teachers' Associations, I have advocated the use of bicarbonate of soda as a preventive for 'Colds,' with the result that now many reports are coming in stating that *those* who took 'Soda' were not affected, while nearly everyone around them had the 'Flu.'

Recommended dosages from the Arm & Hammer Company for colds and influenza back in 1925 were:

- During the first day take six doses of half teaspoonful of Arm & Hammer Bicarbonate of Soda in glass of cool water, at about two hour intervals.

- During the second day take four doses of half teaspoonful of Arm & Hammer Bicarbonate of Soda in glass of cool water, at the same intervals.

- During the third day take two doses of half teaspoonful of Arm & Hammer Bicarbonate of Soda in glass of cool water morning and evening, and thereafter half teaspoonful in glass of cool water each morning until cold is cured.

"Well the sodium bicarbonate cure for colds and sore throats. A friend called as I was reading about it, I told her to try it. She is rapt! Relief in a few hours, and she went to work the following day! And she was miserable and could hardly talk,[3] had just woken with it full on, and was planning on missing work."

This is all very valuable information coming from the Arm & Hammer Baking Soda Company, which sells aluminum-free baking soda. Clearly they knew what they had in their hands 100 years ago; and its long use in medicine sustains the companies published medical views. "Besides doing good in respiratory affections, bicarbonate of soda is of inestimable value in the treatment of Alimentary Intoxication, Pyelitis (inflammation of the pelvis of the kidney), Hyper-Acidity of Urine, Uric Acid disturbances, Rheumatism and Burns. An occasional three-day course of Bicarbonate of Soda increases the alkalinity of the blood, assists elimination and *increases the resisting power of the body to all infectious diseases."*

My father was a veterinarian and as far back as I can remember (I was born in 1938 so my memory goes back to maybe 1943) he would take sodium bicarbonate dissolved in a full glass of warm water whenever he felt a cold coming on. I don't remember him ever coming down with a full-blown cold. He would treat my cold symptoms likewise and I responded equally as well. He also treated farm animals for various illnesses with sodium bicarbonate via a gastric tube and they recovered quickly. So I've known about the benefits of sodium bicarbonate from early childhood on. Glad to see that its benefits are being more widely touted. Although my father was a doctor of veterinarian medicine, he sometimes referred to himself as an MD (Mule Doctor).

Dr. D BW, DO

BICARBONATE AND STOMACH ACID ISSUES

In order to secure the best results with Arm & Hammer Baking Soda when taken internally, certain simple rules must be observed. *MateriaMedica, Pharmacology and Therapeutics* (Bastedo, page 88) clearly outlines these rules to follow:

- The effect of an alkali in the stomach will vary according to the nature of the stomach contents at the time of administration. In the resting period (after food is digested) sodium bicarbonate merely dissolves mucus and is absorbed as bicarbonate into the blood, to increase its alkalinity directly.

- In the digestive period it reduces the secretion of gastric juice, neutralizes a portion of the hydrochloric acid, liberates the carminative carbon dioxide gas, and is absorbed as sodium chloride.

- In cases of fermentation or 'sour stomach' it may neutralize the organic acids and so result in the opening of a spasmodically closed pylorus (the opening between the stomach and the small intestine); while at the same time it acts to overcome flatulency (accumulation of gas in the stomach and bowels). The time of administration must, therefore, be chosen with a definite purpose. Usually for hyperchlorhydria (excess of acid) one hour or two hours after meals will be the period of harmful excess of acid.

- In continuous hyperacidity and in fermentative conditions a dose an hour before meals will tend to prepare the stomach for the next meal; or sometimes a dose will be necessary immediately after eating, because of abnormal acid or base having been present at the commencement of the meal. (For the average person one-half hour after meals is recommended).

- A dose at bedtime tends to check the early morning acidity, or a dose on arising cleans the stomach of acid and mucus before breakfast. Whenever taking a bicarbonate solution internally, the soda should be dissolved in cold water.

In any medical review of sodium bicarbonate we have to pay attention to stomach acid issues. Sodium bicarbonate has a long history of being used as an antacid for short-term relief of stomach upset though this might not necessarily be the best approach to that problem. But it works and does so quickly. The main thrust of this book is not about using bicarbonate for stomach upset and digestion. This chapter does, however, touch on important stomach issues.

People believe that sodium bicarbonate reduces stomach acids and for this reason think that this is not a good idea since stomach acid is crucial for good digestion. The stomach is protected by the epithelial cells, which produce and secrete a bicarbonate-rich solution that coats the mucosa.[4] Bicarbonate is alkaline, a base, and neutralizes the acid secreted by the parietal cells, producing water in the process. This continuous supply of bicarbonate is the main way that our stomach protects itself from auto digestion (the stomach digesting itself) and the overall acidic environment. If one feels that they are deficient in stomach acid one should supplement with hydrochloric acid.

The mucus membrane of the human stomach has 30 million glands which produce gastric juice containing not only acids, but also bicarbonate. The flow of bicarbonate in the stomach amounts from 400 μmol per hour (24.4 mg/h) for a basal output to 1,200 μmol per hour (73.2 mg/h) for a maximal output. Thus at least half a gram of bicarbonate is secreted daily in our stomach. This rate of gastric bicarbonate secretion is 2 to 10 percent of the maximum rate of acid secretion. In the stomach, bicarbonate participates in a mucus-bicarbonate barrier regarded as the first line of the protective and repair mechanisms. On neutralization by acid, carbon dioxide is produced from bicarbonate.[5]

The FDA puts the oral use of sodium bicarbonate as "Generally Recognized as Safe" (GRAS) list and is sold in supermarkets everywhere in the United States with instructions right on the box for oral consumption. It's a food grade item that is generally considered safe with little precautions needed.

Sodium bicarbonate is safe enough to be used with babies and in fact traditional European preparations have used it for centuries to ease the discomforts of infant colic, stomach pain, hiccups, gas, and teething. Such preparations consist of specific herbs known to be beneficial for digestion such as fennel and ginger and a small quantity of sodium bicarbonate.

Ulcers, once thought caused by excess stomach acid, are actually often the result of the H. pylori bacteria, which eats away the stomach lining, making it vulnerable to stomach acid and ulcers. Hydrochloric acid, a strong acid, is one of the compounds that make up the gastric juice. Hydrochloric acid lowers the pH of the stomach contents to sometimes 2.0,[6] providing an extremely acidic environment that kills most microbes in food, including many that could cause human illness. Often what a person has to do to resolve certain digestive and general health problems is to take hydrochloric acid pills to increase stomach acid. Such supplementation can be given with meals if a patient is not capable of reducing heavy protein consumption.

If the acidic contents leaks back into the esophagus, the irritation of the lining there is something we perceive as "heartburn." While most enzymatic digestion occurs in the small intestine, protein digestion begins in the stomach through the action of an enzyme called pepsin. Pepsin is secreted as an inactive material called pepsinogen. The acid environment of the stomach activates it, converting it to pepsin.

Alkaline or acid produced by the body must have an equal and opposite acid or alkaline produced by the body for things to remain in balance. However, alkaline supplied from outside the body, like drinking sodium bicarbonate added to water, results in a net gain of alkalinity in our body. And this is exactly what we want when dealing with most chronic diseases.

Some people are low in stomach acid and then bicarbonate could be balanced with the addition of stomach acids during meals. Dr. Jonathan Wright says that to improve digestion and end heartburn we should increase stomach acid, not decrease it. It is thought that doing so may work by causing the sphincter muscle at the bottom of the esophagus to stay tightly closed in response to the acid in the stomach. It seems that 90 percent of the patients that Dr. Wright tests in his digestion clinic have too little stomach acid, not too much. Dr. Wright prescribes for his patients' hydrochloric acid pills, which he has compounded at compounding pharmacies. One can look for betaine hydrochloride, which is hydrochloric acid in their local health food store as well as pepsin, papaine, bromelian, and pancreatic enzymes, which are what Wright prescribes for his patients.

One of the primary functions of the stomach is to form acid to digest protein, the building blocks of life. Some people might think that taking sodium bicarbonate orally would nullify this effect but that is simply not the case. It is true that the human is an acid consuming, acid metabolizing, acid excreting organism and that is exactly why bicarbonate physiology is so important. Though acid is concentrated especially in the stomach and the bladder in the form of urine, the body in general enjoys life better when we are slightly alkaline. But it is possible to be deficient in stomach acid, which is essential for proper digestion.

Drug companies have been good at creating medications that shut down stomach acid production. Medications like Aciphex, Nexium, Prevacid, Prilosec, and Protonix are among the most frequently prescribed drugs in the country. Prilosec OTC, available without a prescription, has become one of the most popular heartburn pills in the pharmacy. The pharmaceutical industry misses the point badly in directly suppressing acid production.

In reality it's rare to have a case in which a person has too much stomach acid. Most people's problem is stomach acid being excreted at the wrong time, like when there's no food present to use it up. Stressed-out people seem to have more problems with heartburn or acid reflux and it is common to experience flare-ups when emotional.

When it comes to modern western diets heavy with meat, dairy, and quick rising bread even with normal hydrochloric levels people have a difficult time breaking down all the proteins into amino acids, and that is why so many people have difficulties in their intestines to the point of leaking gut syndrome. Sourdough bread is important for this very reason. When bread is digested overnight by natural yeast the proteins get predigested before they ever enter our mouths. This is a central issue with gluten intolerance.

Adding sodium bicarbonate to subjects on a high protein diet, which are known to acidify urine and sometimes lead to hypercalciuria (high level of calcium in urine), has been shown to greatly reduce calcium urinary excretion. The effect has been observed with 5.5 grams of bicarbonate supplement received daily for two weeks. A recent study presented in the review of literature highlights that a bicarbonate-rich mineral water could be useful in the prevention of the recurrence of calcium oxalate and uric acid renal stones.[7]

Stomach acid is actually secreted in reaction to what is put in the mouth. Once nerves in the cheeks and tongue are stimulated by the food, they send messages to the brain, which, in turn, alerts nerves in the stomach wall, stimulating the secretion of gastric juice before the bolus itself arrives in the stomach. Once the bolus touches the stomach lining, it triggers a second release of gastric juice, along with mucus rich in bicarbonate that helps protect the stomach lining from the action of the hydrochloric acid.

When we drink bicarbonate water on an empty stomach it mostly bypasses the stomach acid mechanism because when we drink water or liquids it goes right through the stomach with most liquids being absorbed along the intestinal tract. This fact was observed over 150 years ago when a man was accidentally shot in the stomach.

A Dr. William Beaumont treated his wound, but expected the man to die from his injuries. But the man survived—but with a hole, or fistula, in his stomach that never fully healed. This allowed Dr. Beaumont, and army surgeon, to directly observe the processes of the stomach through many years of research on this particular patient. Liquids are quickly emptied, so baking soda does not have an especially depressing or neutralizing effect on stomach acid especially when taken on an empty stomach.[8] This even happens when we eat, for the water content is wrung out of the food through mechanical action.

> *The cause of "high stomach acid" or ulcers is really Helicobacter Pylori,*
> *which is an acid resistant bacteria, and are killed in presence of sodium bicarbonate.*
> —*Parhatsathid Nabadalung*

The cells in our stomach wall produce hydrochloric acid (HCl) on demand. It is created on an instantly-as-needed basis. The ingredients in the stomach cell that make hydrochloric acid (HCl) are carbon dioxide (CO_2), water (H_2O), and sodium chloride (NaCl) or potassium chloride (KCl).

$$NaCl + H_2O + CO_2 = HCl + NaHCO_3, \text{ or } KCl + H_2O + CO_2 = HCl + KHCO_3$$

The controversy over sodium bicarbonate and its role as a medical treatment might be relatively new, but baking soda has a long history of use. *The Eloquent Peasant,* an Egyptian story that dates to around 2000 BC, refers to a peddler selling natron, a natural blend of sodium bicarbonate, chloride, and sodium carbonate that was used in mummification—just one of hundreds of ways baking soda has been utilized. Baking soda's first widespread use, however, was probably as a leavening agent for bread and other baked goods. It has been used commercially since 1775, although the now-famous Arm & Hammer brand wasn't introduced until 1867.

TREATING RADIOACTIVE, CHEMICAL AND HEAVY METAL TOXICITY

Baking soda lives up to the image on the Arm & Hammer box; it is the ultimate heavyweight workhorse medicine that every healthcare professional and parent should use to diminish toxic poisoning of radiation, heavy metals, and chemicals. The more polluted your environment, the more bicarbonate one needs; it is as simple as that. All men, women and children who live in urban centers become deficient in bicarbonate because bicarbonate is needed to buffer all the acid contaminants. People living/working in a polluted environment have fewer amounts of bicarbonates in their blood than people working in a clean environment.

In the January/February 2003 issue of *American Industrial Hygiene Association Journal,* Dr. Gospodinka R. Pradova published the result of a 10-year study of industrial pollution in Bulgaria. The study compares two groups of people in a plastic manufacturing plant: one group working in the plant with chemical pollution, the other in the non-polluted office environment of the same company. The conclusion shows that people living/working in a polluted environment have *fewer amounts of bicarbonates in their blood* than people working in a clean environment.

So deep are the protective, buffering, and neutralizing properties of bicarbonate that it is used even with radiation exposure to protect the kidneys and other tissues. And in a world that is already overexposed to uranium and mercury, sodium bicarbonate becomes even more important. Because we have built many nuclear plants some of which have melted down with Fukushima showering the world with relentless radiation, every parent has to pay attention because the children are most vulnerable, they need to be protected.

Science already knows that oral administration of sodium bicarbonate as a detox cleanse diminishes the severity of the changes produced by uranium in the kidneys. And it does this for heavy metals and other toxic chemicals, including chemotherapy agents, which are lethal even in low dosages. Since depleted uranium weapons were used starting in the first Gulf War, the United States has polluted the world with uranium oxide and it is showing up more and more in tests doctors perform. With a half-life of several billion years we had better be prepared to get used to dealing with the toxic effects and help our bodies clear it more easily through the kidneys.

Dr. Klinghardt explains the hidden connection between such toxic build up and the inflammatory infections that are principle aspects of heart disease, saying, "Toxic metals harm the cells of the body whereas the invading microorganisms can often thrive in a heavy metal environment. Research by Ludwig, Voll and others in Germany and Omura, and I here in the US show that microorganisms tend to set up their housekeeping in those body compartments that have the highest pollution with toxic metals. The body's own immune cells are incapacitated in those areas whereas the microorganisms multiply and thrive in an undisturbed way." He goes on to suggest that "diagnosing and treating toxic metal residues in the body along with the appropriate treatment of the microorganisms. As long as compartmentalized toxic metals are present in the body, microorganisms have a fortress that cannot be conquered by antibiotics."

What does bicarbonate really do? Baking soda is like a janitor mopping up the messes and carrying the poisons away. This janitor protects tissues and leaves an alkaline film or trail behind to make sure everything stays safe. In medicine, sodium bicarbonate is like the cleaning and security man proven loyal through decades of faithful service and it can be brought in to provide some sort of protection in cases where people are suffering from radiation toxicity.

So useful and strong is sodium bicarbonate that at Los Alamos National Laboratory in New Mexico, researcher Don York has used baking soda to clean soil contaminated with uranium. Sodium bicarbonate binds with uranium, separating it from the dirt; so far, York has removed as much as 92 percent of the uranium from contaminated soil samples.

Medical Officials and the Government Will Not Alert You

The New York Times printed an article recently titled, *Experts Foresee No Detectable Health Impact from Fukushima Radiation.* The UN is concluding that, "It is unlikely to be able to attribute any health effects in the future among the general public and the vast majority of workers." The operator of Japan's crippled Fukushima nuclear plant said on August 23, 2013 that new spots of high radiation levels had been found near storage tanks holding highly contaminated water, raising fear of fresh leaks as the disaster goes from bad to worse. The announcement comes after Tokyo Electric Power Company (Tepco) said already last week that contaminated water with dangerously high levels of radiation was leaking from a storage tank.

Japan's nuclear crisis is escalating! That's really bad news for the human race unless you are one of the many people who believe that nuclear radiation is not a problem. Doctors who use it for diagnosis and treatment believe nuclear radiation is safe enough to use in medicine, but medical science already knows that increasing levels of radiation exposure leads to increases in cancer rates. Oncologists though insist on using something that causes cancer (radiation) to treat it.

Everyone needs to read what *National Geographic* is saying about the rising tensions in Japan as radioactive water leaking into the Pacific Ocean gets dangerously worse. The Japanese government, in August of 2013, is saying that 300 tons (71,895 gallons/272,152 liters) are pouring into the sea each day, enough to fill an olympic-size swimming pool every eight days.

A mathematical model developed by Changsheng Chen of the University of Massachusetts at Dartmouth and Robert Beardsley of the Woods Hole Oceanographic Institute found that radioactive particles disperse through the ocean differently at different depths. The scientists estimated that in some cases, contaminated seawater could reach the western coast of the United States in as little as five years. Buesseler thinks the process occurs a bit more rapidly, and estimates it might take three years for contamination to reach the US coastline. But don't worry. It's not likely to have any real measurable effect on anyone or anything. That is what *Forbes Magazine* would have its readers believe. Reuters is reporting something different though. "The latest leak is so contaminated that a person standing half a meter (1 foot 8 inches) away would, within an hour, receive a radiation dose five times the average annual global limit for nuclear workers. After 10 hours, a worker in that proximity to the leak would develop radiation sickness with symptoms including nausea and a drop in white blood cells.

"That is a huge amount of radiation. The situation is getting worse," said Michiaki Furukawa, who is professor emeritus at Nagoya University and a nuclear chemist. Yuhei Sato, the governor of the Fukushima prefecture in Japan, has described the leak a national emergency. In April, 2013 The Washington Blog reported that:

> A quick calculation shows that it is about ten thousand times less than the amounts released by Chernobyl during the actual fire at the Russian nuclear plant. But the Chernobyl fire only lasted 10 days…and the Fukushima release has been ongoing for more than 2 years so far. Indeed, Fukushima has already spewed much more radioactive cesium and iodine than Chernobyl. The amount of radioactive cesium released by Fukushima was some 20 to 30 times higher than initially admitted. Fukushima also pumped out huge amounts of radioactive iodine 129— which has a half-life of 15.7 million years. Fukushima has also dumped up to 900 trillion becquerels of radioactive strontium-90—which is a powerful internal emitter which mimics calcium and collects in our bones—into the ocean. And the amount of radioactive fuel at Fukushima dwarfs Chernobyl … and so could keep leaking for decades, centuries or millenia.

Radiation at Extremely Low Levels

It is the inability to see the effects of chronic, low level toxicities on human health that has been, and remains, our greatest failing as intelligent beings.
—Dr. Boyd Haley

The world has never awakened to Dr. Haley's warning of many years ago. His warning to the world's scientists and doctors has mostly gone unnoticed meaning we are left with a government, medical officials, and doctors who have no idea of the real dangers people and children are facing as an entire nuclear plant with six reactors is abandoned and goes dangerously out of control.

In July of 2005, the National Academy of Sciences came to the conclusion that the preponderance of scientific evidence shows that even very low doses of radiation pose a risk of cancer or other health problems and there is no threshold below which exposure can be viewed as harmless. *Forbes Magazine's* essay on Fukushima is journalistic trash but what can we expect from beasts in the face of a human nightmare that is promising our children a chilling future.

In the future we are not going to be dealing with radiation at extremely low levels. This past week we learned that deep beneath Fukushima's crippled nuclear power station a massive underground reservoir of contaminated water that began spilling from the plant's reactors after the 2011 earthquake and tsunami has been creeping slowly toward the Pacific sea. Now, $2^1/_2$ years later, experts fear it is about to reach the ocean and greatly worsen what is fast becoming a new crisis at Fukushima, the inability to contain vast quantities of radioactive water.

The looming crisis is potentially far greater than the discovery earlier this week of a leak from a tank that stores contaminated water used to cool the reactor cores. Experts believe the underground seepage from the reactor and turbine building area is much bigger and possibly more radioactive, confronting the plant's operator, Tokyo Electric Power Company, with an invisible, chronic problem and few viable solutions.

"Radiation is continuing to leak out of the reactors, the situation is not stable at all, radiation continues to leak," said Dr. Michio Kaku, professor of theoretical physics at the City University of New York and top graduate of Harvard. "We are looking at a ticking time bomb. It appears stable but the slightest disturbance, a secondary earthquake, a pipe break, evacuation of the crew at Fukushima could set off a full scale meltdown at three nuclear power stations—far beyond what we saw at Chernobyl."

Kaku said this two years ago. The press has been quiet about Fukushima these past two years but things are worsening to the point where events are breaking into the mainstream press. "The Tepco utility people are outclassed and overwhelmed and should be removed from their positions. They are 'making it up as they go along'," Dr. Kaku has said since the beginning, of the efforts of engineers to get this disaster under some control. He also said, "We would see increases in leukemia and thyroid cancers from the massive amounts of radioactive iodine being released."

Recent reports (August 2013) are already showing a disturbing increase in thyroid cancers in the children in the area surrounding Fukushima. The latest figures released by regional authorities brings the total number of children who have been diagnosed with or suspected of having cancer to 44, up from 28 as of June, *The Asahi Shimbun* national daily reports.

> *The average annual rate of childhood leukemia has risen almost*
> *one percent a year from 1977 to 1995.*
> —*National Cancer Institute*

Importance of Bicarbonates

Sodium bicarbonate is useful, not just with radiation but with heavy metals and chemical poisons. Sodium bicarbonate can safely remove paint, grease, oil, and smoke residue, decreasing workers' exposure to harsh chemicals and eliminating much of the hazardous waste associated with other cleaners. "Sodium bicarbonate is able to clean in areas where other substances pose fire hazards because baking soda is a natural fire extinguisher," says Kenneth Colbert, a general manager for Arm & Hammer. This is the reason it's used by oncology centers to control chemo agent spills, and it's actually used intravenously to protect patients from the hazardous toxicity of chemotherapy.

Tissues and cells are like factories with furnace mitochondria everywhere, and everything gets very dirty with acid waste that must be cleared away every millisecond of life. There is no way around the reality that metabolism creates acid waste that can accumulate quite rapidly under the right conditions. Essentially, sodium bicarbonate is a neutralizer of many other compounds, which makes it extremely helpful to the body. Instead of the traditional muscleman with a mallet on Arm & Hammer's baking soda box, a better image might be a janitor sweeping toxins away.

This janitor protects tissues and leaves an alkaline trail behind to make sure everything stays clean. In medicine, sodium bicarbonate is the cleaning agent proven loyal through decades of faithful service.

ORAL HYGIENE

With ample brushing, sodium bicarbonate has the power to break through pathogen films, called biofilms,[9] that sticky stuff that turns into hard tartar that your dentist has to struggle to remove, while you grin and bear it.

Bicarbonate has been shown to decrease dental plaque acidity induced by sucrose, and its buffering capacity plays a major role in preventing dental cavities. Studies have shown that bicarbonate inhibits plaque formation on teeth and, in addition, increases calcium uptake by dental enamel. This effect of bicarbonate on teeth is so well recognized that tooth powder containing sodium bicarbonate was patented in the USA in October 1985.

Sodium bicarbonate has been suggested to increase the pH in the oral cavity, potentially neutralizing the harmful effects of bacterial metabolic

Julia Roberts Uses Sodium Bicarbonate to Brush Her Teeth

Julia Roberts is famous for her bright smile and the actress says she owes it to her grandfather's tip of using baking soda. "I brush [my teeth] with baking soda. [My grandfather] would put a big heaping mound of it on his toothbrush. He had only one cavity in his entire life," Roberts said.

Her grandfather was around in the early days of medicine when sodium bicarbonate made by the Arm & Hammer Baking Soda Company was in its heyday publishing about how baking soda can be used as a medicine. Yes it keeps her teeth white, but it does much more than that. Sodium bicarbonate, used in more and more toothpastes and in the newer dental teeth-cleaning devices, is the very best agent for the maintenance of oral health because it changes pH, radically disrupting the constantly rising tide of bacteria and fungi that threaten the health status of the entire body.

acids. Sodium bicarbonate is increasingly used in dentistry and its presence appears to be less abrasive to enamel and dentine than other commercial toothpastes.

Why Is This Important?

Through the years scientists have discovered a conclusive link between gum disease and both cancer and heart disease. "Our study provides the first strong evidence that *periodontal disease increases the risk of pancreatic cancer,*" said Dr. Dominique Michaud of the Harvard School of Public Health in Boston, who led the research. Men with a history of periodontal disease *had a 64 percent increased risk of pancreatic cancer* than men with no such history.

People with increased severity of periodontitis with recent tooth loss had the greatest risk. People with periodontal disease have an increased level of inflammatory markers such as C-reactive protein (CRP) in their blood. These markers are part of an early immune system response to persistent inflammation and have been linked to the development of pancreatic cancer. It is the high levels of carcinogenic compounds that are present in the mouths of people with periodontal disease that increases risk of pancreatic cancer.[10]

> ***Most of our cancer patients have a lot of amalgam dental fillings.***
> *—Professor W. Kostler, President of Austrian Society of Oncology*

Mercury vapors in the mouth, increased use of antibiotics, periodontal disease, inappropriate oral care, yeast and fungal overgrowth, and decreasing immune strength are all colliding and reinforcing each other in a downward spiral that leads to chronic diseases and cancer. *More than 50 million Americans suffer from periodontitis.*

The underlying causes of periodontal disease are infectious agents such as virus, bacteria, spirochetes, amoebas, and fungus. Periodontitis is a micro climate that reflects the macro climate of the entire body. A published study in the *Journal of Periodontology* confirms recent findings that people with periodontal disease are at a greater risk of systemic diseases, and periodontal disease appears to be a risk factor for heart disease and stroke. Men with periodontitis had a 72 percent greater risk of developing coronary disease. Gingivitis was associated with a 42 percent increased risk for men. A 1996 study involving over 1,100 individuals found that the incidence of coronary heart disease, fatal coronary disease, and strokes were all significantly related to their baseline periodontal status.[11]

In periodontal disease the pathogens form of a sticky, colorless plaque that constantly forms on our teeth, however other factors can cause periodontal (gum) disease or influence its progression. Harvard Medical School researchers studied longevity and found that one of the most important factors for prevention of periodontal disease and gingivitis is daily flossing, because it removes bacteria from the teeth and gums.

As the plaque gets harder and thicker, it becomes what is known as dental calculus or tartar, a hard calcified layer that is virtually impossible to shift with normal brushing, you would have to get the dental hygienist to do it. Gingivitis is the inflammation of the gums around the teeth due in great part to improper cleaning of the teeth. Although systemic factors and general health can modify the tissue reactions to local irritants, the primary irritant is mercury-containing dental amalgam.

> *The Richardson Report, a study completed for Canada health in 1995, found that the tolerable daily intake of mercury was exceeded in different age groups with the following number of amalgam fillings: adults—4, teenager—3, children and toddlers—1.*
> *—Dr. Robert Gammal*

Scientific Findings

Several studies have found a strong relationship between the bacterium causing gum disease and atherosclerosis. In fact, the same bacterium that has been cultured from the crud, or plaque, is seen in arteries. According to an article published in the *Archives of Otolaryngology—Head and Neck Surgery*, chronic periodontitis is associated with an increased risk of developing cancer of the tongue among men.[12] Researchers at the University at Buffalo and Roswell Park Cancer Institute have found the same thing.

> *Periodontal disease has increased prevalence amongst patients with certain systemic diseases such as type-2 diabetes mellitus.[13]*

Oral candidiasis, a fungal infection in the mouth, appears more frequent amongst diabetics and people who wear dentures. If you smoke, have high blood glucose levels or take antibiotics often, you are more likely to have a problem with oral fungal infections. Oral candidiasis is also more common amongst immunocompromised people such as those that have HIV or AIDS, are pregnant, or are undergoing chemotherapy or radiation therapy.

The incidence of oral cancer is on the rise. Current estimates have the rate of increase at around 11percent, with approximately 34,000 people in the US being diagnosed with oral cancers each year. Of those 34,000 newly diagnosed individuals, only half will be alive in five years. Oral cancer can mimic common mouth sores meaning most patients do not experience noticeable symptoms in the early stage of the disease process, and that is dangerous.

Stop using floridated toothpaste! Commercial toothpastes are worthless as healing oral health agents though it does take a serious adjustment of the mind to throw out those tubes that have been around since we could walk and talk.

> *Sodium bicarbonate is used to reduce the inflammation of oral mucosa resulting from chemotherapeutic agents or ionizing radiation. Mucositis typically manifests as erythema or ulcerations.[14]*

7. *Sodium Bicarbonate and Cancer*

On January 3rd of 2013 medical scientists published, "The results of a study suggesting that tumor cells do, indeed, perform niche engineering by creating an acidic environment that is non-toxic to the malignant cells but, through its negative effects on normal cells and tissue, promotes local invasion." A number of studies have shown that the extracellular pH in cancers is typically lower than that in normal tissue and that an acidic pH promotes invasive tumor growth in primary and metastatic cancers. The external pH of solid tumors is acidic as a consequence of increased metabolism of glucose and poor perfusion. Acid pH has been shown to stimulate tumor cell invasion and metastasis *in vitro* and in cells before tail vein injection *in vivo*.

Researchers have investigated the very reasonable assumption that increased systemic concentrations of pH buffers would lead to reduced intratumoral and peritumoral acidosis and, as a result, inhibit malignant growth. Researchers have also found that consequent reduction of tumor acid concentrations significantly reduces tumor growth and invasion without altering the pH of blood or normal tissues.[1]

Scientific Findings

Dr. Robert J. Gillies and team from Wayne State University School of Medicine published a paper entitled, *Acidity generated by the tumor microenvironment drives local invasion.* Gillies and his colleagues have demonstrated that pre-treatment of mice with sodium bicarbonate results in the alkalization of the area around tumors. The same researchers reported that bicarbonate increases tumor pH and also inhibits spontaneous metastases in mice with breast cancer.[2] It also reduces the rate of lymph node involvement.

Bicarbonate has been found to "enhance the anti-tumor activity" of other anticancer drugs. This is similar to recently published research about injecting O_2 directly into tumors where such direct administration of oxygen also facilitated the action of chemotherapy.

What researchers are finding makes sense. Areas of tumor with the lowest pH (greatest acidity) have the highest invasiveness. Thus when scientists neutralized the acidity with oral sodium bicarbonate, the invasion was halted. By simply changing the pH with baking soda they turned invasive cancers into retreating cancers.

Tumor cells behave like any plant or animal in altering the local environment to promote its own survival. Cancers are literally invading species in our body and that is why Dr. Simoncini is not wrong when he claims cancer is a fungus. We will spend several chapters talking about this and the late stage fungus infections most late stage cancer patients suffer from.

No matter what we believe the cells to be we know without doubt that tumor cells metabolize glucose at high rates and this creates a lot of acid. The tumor cells adapt and bathe themselves in this high acid–low oxygen situation. They love it, but the surrounding cells don't. The tumor cells are altering their local environment to ensure their own survival and the death of tissues that surround the tumors. The high-acid environment leads to a cascade of problems, which can all be piled together to contribute to the rotting of healthy tissues. Normal cells die, and cancer can expand and invade more and more territory. I recently received this letter from a doctor.

I am a Surgeon practicing in South America. I have been using $NaHCO_3$ in my patients with Prostate Cancer Stage 4. The results have been quite amazing. The only available form of NaHC03 is baking soda (Arm & Hammer). I chose the Prostate Cancer cases Stage 4 since those cases are practically beyond the capacity of surgery to manage except for bilateral Orchidectomy. Patients can't afford all the other drugs for Chemical Castration so I have performed Surgical Castration (Orchidectomy) before I read of $NaHCO_3$. I check their PSA before giving them $NaHCO_3$ and monitor the PSA monthly thereafter. I also do the usual Rectal Exam, Ultra Sound, Pelvic and Spine X-rays and CT scan if patients can afford it. Since the measuring teaspoon is not always available I use the ordinary teaspoon. The dose I use is one level teaspoon twice daily in a glass of water with one teaspoon honey to make it more palatable. I tried it myself for the past two years now just to see what effect it gives to me and for pro-phylaxis. Surprisingly my backache due to Ankylosing Spondylitis have vir-tually disappeared, which I never expected. Recently I was able to get hold of the tablet form preparation, 325 mgs, which I substituted instead of baking soda because of the ease in which to take it. Is this as effective? I noticed that using the baking soda at the dose above I would burp after a few minutes like when drinking a carbonated drink, but this does not happen when I use the tablet form. The PSA of all patients I gave NaHC03 have gone down to normal in almost all cases while a few are just slightly above 10. One patient had a PSA of 297 and after 6 months of NaHC03 the PSA came down to 11.1. I expect it to be normal in a month.

Sincerely, MNF

University of Arizona Cancer Center member Dr. Mark Pagel received a 2 million dollar grant from the National Institutes of Health to study the effectiveness of baking soda therapy to treat breast cancer. He wrote that his "Research focuses on pre-clinical studies in a laboratory setting. More importantly, my research primarily focuses on the refinement of my method for measuring tumor acidosis using non-invasive magnetic resonance imag-ing methods. One application of this method is to monitor changes in acid content (pH) in tumors and normal tissues following baking soda treat-ment. But there are other applications as well. For example, tumor acidosis causes chemo-resistance to common anti-cancer drugs such as doxorubicin and paclitaxel. Determining whether an individual's tumor is acidic can aid in selecting the appropriate chemotherapy for that individual patient, lead-ing to "personalized medicine." Dr. Pagel said, "Furthermore, there is some evidence that pH-neutral tumors do NOT respond well to baking soda treatment. This is plausible because tumors that are not acidic don't need to be neutralized by baking soda (however, this preliminary evidence is not yet proof that pH-neutral tumors will not respond to baking soda treat-ment). Thus, a patient may have a pH-neutral tumor and experience no ben-efit from baking soda, and yet take too much baking soda for too long and cause damage to normal tissues. That would be unacceptable. This concern that normal tissues may become alkalinized provides additional justifica-tion for developing a non-invasive imaging method to monitor pH through-out the body."

Importance of Bicarbonates

The justification for using bicarbonate does not center solely on its pH tumor controlling or reducing role. If a person is bicarbonate deficient, too acidic, and if the deficiency is addressed, the entire body including the immune system will work better and this helps in cancer treatment. Everyone's bicarbonate level declines with age and it would be quite unusual to find a cancer patient without a generalized bicarbonate deficiency no matter what the pH of the tumors are. If there are tumors that are actually alkaline it would indeed be a rare condition because the respiration of cancer cells creates acid conditions.

There is no hiding the fact that baking soda, the same stuff that can save a person's life in the emergency room in a heartbeat, is a primary cancer treatment option of the safest most effective kind. I never suggest though that it should be used out of the context of a full cancer protocol of medicinals that support bicarbonate's cancer eliminating role.

To depend on baking soda or anything else as a sole cancer cure is misguided and risky. But when used as a primary anti-cancer agent with other anti-cancer agents it is intelligent. When taken orally with water, especially water with high magnesium content, and when used transdermally in medicinal baths, baking soda becomes a first-line medicinal for the treatment of cancer.

One does not have to be a doctor to practice pH medicine. Every practitioner of the healing arts and every mother and father needs to understand how to use sodium bicarbonate.

> *Virtually all degenerative diseases including cancer, heart disease, arthritis, osteoporosis, kidney and gall stones, and tooth decay are associated with excess acidity in the body.*

There is nothing that will make aggressive metastatic cells more aggressive than having acid conditions ruling over the body. The right conditions in the body will enable cancer cells to grow faster and more robustly, but nothing will cut the rug from under cancer cells faster than sodium bicarbonate, which very quickly changes the basic terrain that cancers grow in. Baking soda (sodium bicarbonate) replaces much harsher chemo agents and radiation therapy and even surgery can be avoided when we literally cut the legs out from cancer cells by rapidly changing the pH environment.

Bicarbonate and Rapid pH Shifts

Sodium bicarbonate is safe, extremely inexpensive, and effective when it comes to cancer tissues. It is irresistible cyanide to cancer cells. It hits the cancer cells with a shock wave of alkalinity, which allows much more oxygen into the cancer cells than they can tolerate. Cancer cells cannot survive in the presence of high levels of oxygen. Sodium bicarbonate is, for all intent and purposes, a quick killer of tumors.

Every cancer patient should know that oral intake of sodium bicarbonate offers a strong shift of body pH into the alkaline. So strong is the effect that athletes can notice the difference in their breathing as more oxygen (and thus CO_2) is carried throughout the system, as more acids are neutralized.[3] The difference can be stunning for those whose respiration is labored under intense exercise loading.[4]

Bicarbonates action is immediate. As a cancer treatment a course of treatment runs about two weeks, which can be repeated over and over again. Bicarbonate, when used in conjunction with other equally safe substances, can form the basis for a natural chemotherapy.

In the case of sodium bicarbonate, we have common sense biochemistry at work. Sodium bicarbonate possesses the property of absorbing heavy metals, dioxins, and furans. Comparison of cancer tissue with healthy tissue from the same person shows that the cancer tissue has a much higher concentration of toxic materials, such as chemicals, and pesticides.

Diagnosing Cancer with Bicarbonate Physiology

Orthodox oncologists have had much to learn about bicarbonate and now are finding out that bicarbonate can even be used to diagnose cancer in its earliest stages. We know that bicarbonate turns to CO_2 easily when dissolved in water as it enters the stomach, but few know that cancerous tissue turns bicarbonate into carbon dioxide. A few years ago, a United Kingdom Cancer Research team found MRI scans were able to track changes in bicarbonate and therefore identify cancers even in the very early stages.

All cancer has a lower pH, meaning it is more acidic than surrounding tissue. Working with mice, the researchers boosted the MRI sensitivity more than 20,000 times. Using MRI, they looked to see how much of the tagged bicarbonate was converted into carbon dioxide within the tumor. In more acidic tumors, more bicarbonate is converted into carbon dioxide.

Lead researcher Professor Kevin Brindle, from Cancer Research UK's Cambridge Research Institute at the University of Cambridge, said, "This technique could be used as a highly-sensitive early warning system for the signs of cancer. By exploiting the body's natural pH balancing system, we have found a potentially safe way of measuring pH to see what's going on inside patients. MRI can pick up on the abnormal pH levels found in cancer, and it is possible that this could be used to pinpoint where the disease is present and when it is responding to treatment."

8. *Cancer Treatment Philosophy*

Imagine your cancer cells being caught between a brutal crossfire. Military personnel understand war tactics and how to best capture the enemy in a trap from which there is no escape. Natural Allopathic Medicine is introducing to the world an aggressive nontoxic method of winning the war against cancer, offering new tactics and combining them with some very successful old ones.

Cancer is a prime example of how heavy metal toxicity, free radical damage, pathogen infection, inflammation, mitochondria dysfunction, immune system depression, mineral and vitamin deficiencies, genetic mutation, cell wall damage, and oxidative stress all come together into an end-stage, life-threatening condition. Cancer treatment can be approached in many ways, but the best way is to address all these problems simultaneously.

Everyone wants to maximize their chances of recovering from cancer and this is accomplished first by understanding the idea of using a protocol of anti-cancer agents, each part delivering heavy duty medical firepower. By overlapping zones of fire (pharmacological effects) we raise the rate by which we will see positive therapeutic effect meaning, complete cure or remission of cancerous conditions. Natural Allopathic Medicine's protocol traps cancer tumors/cells in a lethal fire of concentrated nutritional substances.

Calling in the Best Armor Divisions

Any general would be more than thrilled to have an army of medicinals at his disposal that cause severe difficulties for the enemy (unhealthy cells turned cancerous and proliferating infections) while being extremely friendly to one's own troop of cells. It is a disaster in war when friendly fire falls on one's own troops (cells) and this is exactly what happens in orthodox cancer treatments, which are so toxic they can kill the host too. Chemotherapy wipes out the enemy, but at the price of killing friendly healthier cells. Chemotherapy's agents are blunt instruments—toxins that kill healthy cells just as effectively as they kill cancer cells. Because nutritional medicine is nontoxic in nature, we can layer treatments and attack from all sides in a simultaneous assault on cancer that is dead set on taking our life.

It is no longer appropriate to consider drugs or nutritional medical agents in isolation. Protocols entail combining substances that have not been tested together, but have been individually proven to be effective. This combination or protocol approach is theoretically impossible with pharmaceutical drugs because it is impossible to predict how toxic chemicals and poisons (drugs) will mix together.

It rarely happens that one medicine or medical treatment conclusively resolves a serious chronic medical problem. It is generally a mistake to try to isolate drugs the way the pharmaceutical companies do and pin the hopes of millions on a single medication. Yet companies that produce and market their health products clearly isolate their solutions trying the best they can to induce people in their direction. A focus on combination therapy enables us to encompass and manage multiple risk factors. Multidimensional etiologies call for multiple therapeutic interventions.

Extracellular Matrix Regulates Gene Expression and Cancer

Gene mutations are part of the process of cancer, but *mutations alone are not enough to cause cancer* to take hold and spread; thus threatening people's lives through domination of precious life resources (nutrition) as well as precious real estate where other healthy cells live. Genes do become damaged and sustain mutations in some cells and not others during people's lifetimes. An oncogene—a gene that causes tumors in animals and uncontrolled growth in cells in culture—cannot in and of itself change cells from normal to cancerous. It is the cells' surroundings, known as its *microenvironment*, that contribute in some way to how cancer has occurred.

Cancer involves an interaction between rogue cells and surrounding tissue. This is the clear message that Dr. Mina Bissell, who is the director of life sciences at the Lawrence Berkeley National Lab in California (LBNL), and she is now sharing this with the world. The interactions between cancer cells and their *micro* and *macroenvironment* create a context that promotes tumor growth and protects them from immune attack or, on the other hand, prevent tumors from making any kind of beachhead so they cannot take hold or spread themselves around. Cancer cells routinely form in most people's bodies, but that does not mean they are going to succeed in capturing their host's valuable resources so they can invade (inland so to speak) as they win their war and take our life.

What this means is that the surrounding cells and the surrounding extracellular matrix interact to shape cancer cell behaviors such as polarity, migration, and proliferation. The microenvironment includes complex scaffolding on which cells grow and develop, called the extracellular matrix. The microenvironment is what actually surrounds a cell. The extracellular matrix (microenvironment) has been shown to regulate gene expression so it has more to do with the state of cancer than the cancer cells themselves. "If tissue architecture and context are part of the message, then tumor cells with abnormal genomes should be capable of becoming 'normal,'" if grown in a healthy microenvironment. She and her students tested that hypothesis with some malignant cells, growing them on healthy scaffolding. And yes, they were able to revert the malignant phenotype to a normal one. They could even inject the cells into mice where they didn't cause tumors, unlike malignant cells, which would cause cancer. This, says Bissell, indicates that there is another way to look at cancer—that cancer genes are regulated by the environment around them.

Dr. Bissell's basic idea is that cancer cells cannot turn into a lethal tumor without the cooperation of other cells nearby. It is not just the other surrounding cells, but also the interstitial environment, which of course would include pH and nutrient levels being supplied by the blood. That may be why autopsies repeatedly find that most people who die of causes other than cancer have at least some tiny tumors in their bodies that had gone unnoticed. According to current thinking, the tumors were kept in check, causing no harm.

"Think of it as this kid in a bad neighborhood," said Dr. Susan Love, a breast cancer surgeon and president of the Dr. Susan Love Research Foundation. "You can take the kid out of the neighborhood and put him in a different environment and he will behave totally differently." She added, "It's exciting. What it means, if all these environmental findings are right, is that we should be able to reverse cancer without having to kill cells. This could open up a whole new way of thinking about cancer that would be much less assaultive." Dr. Bissell is now hailed as a hero, with an award named after her. "You have created a paradigm shift," the Federation of American Societies for Experimental Biology wrote in a letter announcing that she had won its 2008 Excellence in Science award. Nothing will change a cells environment quicker than sodium bicarbonate.

Scientific Findings—Chemotherapy Provokes More Not Less Cancer

Chemotherapy can cause damage to healthy cells which triggers them to secrete a protein that sustains tumor growth and makes cancer more resistance to any further treatment. We are beginning to see clinical evidence across the board show that what happens to healthy cells during cancer treatment determines much if not the entire outcome of treatment.

"Cancer cells inside the body live in a very complex environment or neighborhood. Where the tumor cell resides and who its neighbors are influence its response and resistance to therapy," said senior author Dr. Peter S. Nelson, a member of the Hutchinson Cancer Center's Human Biology Division. "Our findings indicate that the tumor microenvironment also can influence the success or failure of these more precise therapies." In other words, the same cancer cell, when exposed to different "neighborhoods," may have very different responses to treatment.

Researchers at the Center tested the effects of a type of chemotherapy on tissue collected from men with prostate cancer, and found "evidence of DNA damage" in healthy cells after treatment, they reported in Nature Medicine in August of 2012. The scientists found that healthy cells damaged by chemotherapy secreted more of a protein called WNT16B which boosts cancer cell survival. The researchers observed up to 30-fold increases in WNT production! "The increase in WNT16B was completely unexpected," said Dr. Nelson. The protein was taken up by tumor cells neighboring the damaged cells. "WNT16B, when secreted, would interact with nearby tumor cells and cause them to grow, invade, and importantly, resist subsequent therapy," said Nelson. Rates of tumor cell reproduction have been shown to accelerate between chemotherapy treatments. "Our results indicate that damage responses in benign cells . . . may directly contribute to enhanced tumor growth kinetics," wrote the team. The researchers said they confirmed their findings with breast and ovarian cancer tumors. Dr. Nelson describes the normal insanity/methods of chemotherapy saying, "In the laboratory we can 'cure' most any cancer simply by giving very high doses of toxic therapies to cancer cells in a petri dish. However, in people, these high doses would not only kill the cancer cells, but also normal cells and the host." Therefore, treatments for common solid tumors are given in smaller doses and in cycles, or intervals, to allow the normal cells to recover. This approach may not eradicate all of the tumor cells, and those that survive can evolve to become resistant to subsequent rounds of anti-cancer therapy.

Researchers questioning people who were going through chemotherapy for cancer find the majority—72 percent—experience side effects.[1] The side effect of the Natural Allopathic protocol for cancer is limited to making people feel better. It might not save every patient's life, for often the damage from radiation, chemotherapy, and surgery is too great. Dr. Martin Scurr asks why doctors, like himself, would rather die than endure the pain of treatment for advanced cancer saying, "Some doctors have admitted they wouldn't have the operations they recommend to terminally ill patients. Like most doctors, I understand that much of the care we offer patients who have serious, life-threatening illness is ultimately futile. Worse, it can involve many months of grueling treatments that might possibly extend the length of one's life, but do nothing for the quality. But while we give that care to patients, the vast majority of doctors I know would not want this for themselves."[2]

What mainstream researchers are failing to find is that we can approach cancer treatment from a completely different and opposite angle to chemotherapy. Instead of trying to kill the cancer and harm the surrounding cells, we imprison the cancer in a solid wall of healthy cells, that area being strengthened as opposed to weakened by treatments. We create the conditions where we first limit the ability to grow and then send in some cruise missiles that directly target the cancer cells, choking the life out of them with waves of increased alkalinity and oxygen.

Radiation Medicine and Sodium Bicarbonate

Dr. Edward Golembe, who directs a hyperbaric oxygen chamber at Brookdale University Hospital in Brooklyn, said he had treated serious radiation injuries to the jaw and called them "a horrible, horrible thing to see." When we deal with radiation, we deal with death. It is the death principle that doctors are trying to harness with terrible results. Most people who employ radiation in their treatments for cancer suffer horribly but some worse than others.

Just being alive today is to walk through the valley and shadow of death in terms of radiation exposure. Background radiation on earth has increased in the nuclear age coming from all the above ground testing of the last century, nuclear plants, nuclear waste, uranium mining, and from depleted uranium weapons that are commonly used in the American, British and Israeli armies, navies, and air forces. In addition there is constant and increasing exposure to other forms of radiation from microwave towers, cell phones, wireless phones, and computer systems.

And if that were not enough, the medical establishment throws all caution to the wind and subjects more and more people to higher and higher levels of radiation with medical testing. The late Dr. John W. Gofman, former Professor Emeritus of Molecular and Cell Biology at the University of

California, Berkeley, estimated that about three-quarters of all breast cancer cases in the United States are induced by radiation—including medical X-rays, and including mammograms to detect breast cancer.[3]

So deep are the protective, buffering, and neutralizing properties of bicarbonate that it is used even with radiation exposure to protect the kidneys and other tissues. In a world that is already overexposed to uranium and mercury, sodium bicarbonate becomes even more important because mercury and uranium oxide directly attack the nuclear material and mitochondria of the cells.

The oral administration of sodium bicarbonate diminishes the severity of the changes produced by uranium in the kidneys.[4]The kidneys are usually the first organs to show chemical damage upon uranium exposure. Old military manuals suggest doses or infusions of sodium bicarbonate to help alkalinize the urine if this happens. This makes the uranyl ion less kidney-toxic and promotes excretion of the nontoxic uranium-carbonate complex. The oral administration of sodium bicarbonate diminishes the severity of the changes produced by uranium in the kidneys.[5]

It does this for all the heavy metals and other toxic chemicals including chemotherapy agents, which are highly lethal even in low dosages. After depleted uranium weapons were used starting in the first Gulf War, the United States has polluted the world with uranium oxide and it is showing up more and more in tests doctors perform. With a half-life of several billion years, we had better be prepared to get used to dealing with the toxic effects and help our bodies clear it more easily through the kidneys. Sodium bicarbonate is an absolute must item in any field hospital, and it should be in used and recommended in all clinics and be present in every home medicine cabinet.

So useful and strong is sodium bicarbonate that at Los Alamos National Laboratory in New Mexico, researcher Don York has used baking soda to clean soil contaminated with uranium. *Sodium bicarbonate binds with uranium,* separating it from the dirt; so far, York has removed as much as 92 percent of the uranium from contaminated soil samples. I started writing about baking soda after discovering that the United States Army recommends the use of bicarbonate to protect the kidneys from radiation damage.

Blaise W. LeBlanc, a former research chemist with the US Department of Agriculture, identified the byproduct hydroxymethylfurfural (HMF) as a potential culprit in colony collapse disorder of bees. LeBlanc has a solution to minimize HMF toxicity: By adding bases (such as sodium bicarbonate, or baking soda, lime, potash, or caustic soda) to HFCS, the *pH rises and HMF levels drop.* Sodium bicarbonate can safely remove paint, grease, oil, and smoke residue, decreasing workers' exposure to harsh chemicals and eliminating much of the hazardous waste associated with other cleaners.

"Sodium bicarbonate is able to clean in areas where other substances pose fire hazards, because baking soda is a natural fire extinguisher," says Kenneth Colbert, a general manager for Arm & Hammer. This is the reason it's used by oncology centers to control chemo agent spills, and its actually used intravenously to protect patients from the hazardous toxicity of chemotherapy.

Treating the Underlying Causes of Cancer

The principal lesson to learn for anyone facing cancer is that there are many ways to kill cancer cells and get the body back in balance. What all cancer patients need to understand is that nothing will heal or actually cure cancer until we address and treat the underlying cause of the cancer. The problem here is that there is a complexity of causes. They are layered one on top of the other, so it is not exactly easy to identify the principle cause in each case and not always easy to address it in an appropriate way.

"Cancer is a systemic, not a localized, disease; it is a warning from your body that your diet and lifestyle need to be changed. Eighty percent of your genetic predisposition towards disease can either be activated or held in check by proper diet and lifestyle. Every one of us has some cancer cells in our body every day, and our immune system is usually successful in destroying it; so a strong immune system is a key to fighting cancer. We only notice cancer if it overwhelms our immune system and grows into a noticeable tumor. Even when you've beaten cancer, it is important to maintain a healthy diet and lifestyle so that you won't get it back, especially since you already know that you have a tendency to get cancer. In one study, they found live breast cancer cells still circulating in people who were pronounced 'cured' seven or more years later! This emphasizes the importance of taking care of ourselves even after we're cured," writes Dr. Charles Morris.

Dr. Artour Rakhimov says, "It is not oxygen, but carbon dioxide that is the substance responsible for the main improvement in oxygenation of tissues. Dissolved baking soda has only one effect on composition of arterial blood; it increases its CO_2 content. CO_2, as many medical studies proved, is a powerful vasodilator. It expands arteries and arterioles leading to the tumor since these blood vessels have layers of smooth muscles sensitive to CO_2." Thus sodium bicarbonate addresses cancer tumors in a two prong attack. It increases pH, which in and of itself brings more O_2 to the tissues, while it increases perfusion of blood into the tumors via vasodilation.

Professor Ian Tannock and his colleagues at the University of Toronto have written, "Solid tumors have been observed to develop an acidic extra-cellular environment." This "is believed to occur as a result of lactic acid accumulation produced during aerobic and anaerobic glycolysis." However, these authors also point out that lactic acid production is "not the only mechanism responsible for the development of an acidic environment within solid tumors" (Newell, 1993). Another mechanism might be the poor perfusion of blood around tumors (Robey, 2009).

A large group of British scientists from the Paul Strickland Scanner Centre revealed that when 14 cancer patients breathed various carbogen mixtures (with 2 percent, 3.5 percent, and 5 percent CO_2 content, the rest was O_2) "arterial oxygen tension increased at least three-fold from basal values." (Baddeley et al, 2000) Another group of British researchers directly measured oxygen pressure in cancer cells and concluded, "This study confirms that breathing 2 percent CO_2 and 98 percent O_2 is well tolerated and effective in increasing tumor oxygenation." (Powell et al, 1999)

When it comes to sodium bicarbonate therapy for cancer some think that, "Relying on this type of treatment alone and avoiding or delaying conventional medical care for cancer may have serious health consequences." In this book it is stressed that sodium bicarbonate should not be used alone, but within the context of a full protocol. It is belittling to medical intelligence to conceptualize one individual medicinal as a cancer cure since there are literally hundreds of such medicinal, but some are much stronger than others.

9. Bicarbonate CO_2 Medicine

The co-star of this book is carbon dioxide (CO_2) because bicarbonate and CO_2 are different forms of the same thing. We could have called this book *CO_2 Medicine*. When we talk about bicarbonate we are talking about CO_2. That is what sodium bicarbonate turns to when it reaches the stomach causing an increase in stomach acid production as well as an increase in bicarbonates in the blood. Bicarbonate is an important buffer essential to balanced blood chemistry.

The bicarbonate ion is HCO_3^-. Carbon dioxide is present in the blood in a number of forms such as bicarbonate, dissolved carbon dioxide, and carbonic acid, out of which 90 percent is bicarbonate or HCO_3. The rapid and direct inter-conversion of dissolved CO_2 and bicarbonate ion is catalyzed by the enzyme carbonic anhydrase. Understanding of this relationship between CO_2 and bicarbonate is the key to understanding health and medicine.

"Carbon dioxide is, in fact, a more fundamental component of living matter than is oxygen. Life probably existed on earth for millions of years prior to the carboniferous era, in an atmosphere containing a much larger amount of carbon dioxide than at present. There may even have been a time when there was no free oxygen available in the air," wrote Dr. Yandell Henderson from the *Cyclopedia of Medicine* in 1940. He also said, "Carbon dioxide is the chief hormone of the entire body; it is the only one that is produced by every tissue and that probably acts on every organ."

Henderson exposes why sodium bicarbonate works so dramatically the way it does. According to Henderson, carbon dioxide exerts at least three well-defined influences:

1. It is one of the prime factors in the acid-base balance of the blood.

2. It is the principal control of respiration.

3. It exerts an essential tonic influence upon the heart and peripheral circulation.

Scientific Findings

Dr. Alina Vasiljeva and Dr. David Nias wrote, "At the end of the 19th century, scientists Bohr and Verigo discovered what seemed a strange law: a decreased level of carbon dioxide in the blood leads to decreased oxygen supply to the cells in the body such as the brain, heart, and kidneys. Carbon dioxide (CO_2) was found to be responsible for the bond between oxygen and hemoglobin.

In the 19th century, Zuntz, in Berlin, recognized that carbon dioxide, unlike oxygen, is not carried by hemoglobin. He showed that, in the blood, carbon dioxide is combined with bases, chiefly as sodium bicarbonate which plays a part in acid-alkaline balance. All the carbon dioxide is dissolved in the plasma, both in simple solution and that combined with alkali into the bicarbonates.

If the level of carbon dioxide in the blood is lower than normal, then this leads to difficulties in releasing oxygen from hemoglobin; hence the Verigo-Bohr law. "When we finally come to understand that CO_2 is as much a human food as it is food for plants, meaning its essential for healthy life, no sooner will we understand sodium bicarbonate and why it is so helpful to us when we are confronted with major diseases like cancer, diabetes, neurological, kidney, and Lyme diseases.

Baking soda (sodium bicarbonate) immediately reacts when it mixes with stomach acid.

$$NaHCO_3 + HCl \longrightarrow NaCl + H_2O + CO_2.$$

That is: Sodium bicarbonate + stomach acid yields salt + water + carbon dioxide.

The change of pH value causes the stomach to produce hydrochloric acid that enters the stomach, and the bicarbonates enter the bloodstream. Carbon dioxide is a neutral, nonpolar molecule, and can readily diffuse across membranes. Bicarbonate is a charged species of CO_2, and does not cross membranes at a significant rate unless facilitated by trans-membrane channels like the magnesium calcium channel.

Mix sodium bicarbonate in a bath with lots of citric acid and presto one has a chemical reaction that creates trillions of micro bubbles of CO_2, which will diffuse easily across skin membranes. The bicarbonate ion is amphoteric, meaning that it can behave as either an acid or a base, depending on what it reacts with.

If a bicarbonate ion is combined with an acid, then it behaves as a base.

$$H^+ + HCO_3^- \Longleftrightarrow H_2O + CO_2$$

. . . and carbon dioxide is liberated.

If bicarbonate is combined with a base, then it behaves as an acid 83

$$OH^- + HCO_3^- \Longleftrightarrow HOH + CO_3$$

We normally think of it as a base because it raises the pH of water by accepting a proton:

$$HCO_3^- + H_2O \Longleftrightarrow H2CO_3 + OH^-$$

But if you add bicarbonate to a strongly basic solution, it actually lowers the pH by donating a proton.

$$HCO_3^- + OH^- <==> CO_3\,(_2^-) + H_2O$$

According to the Verigo-Bohr effect, a CO_2 deficit caused by over-breathing leads to partial oxygen starvation in the cells of the body. This state is known as hypoxia (oxygen deficiency), and it negatively affects the nervous system.

Joseph Priestley observed in 1775 that "a green matter" deposited on the walls of water containers, formed bubbles of pure "dephlogisticated air" (oxygen) (Priestley, 1776). While Ingen-Housz (1779, 1796) discovered the importance of light in this process; it was Senebier (1782) who demonstrated that *the production of oxygen by plants depends on the presence of CO_2.*

Oxygen and carbon dioxide are not antagonistic. A gain of one gas in the blood does not necessarily involve a corresponding loss of the other. The blood may be high or low in both gases. Under clinical conditions, low oxygen and low carbon dioxide generally occur together. Therapeutic increase of carbon dioxide, by inhalation of this gas diluted in air, is often an effective means of improving the oxygenation of the blood and tissues.[1]

People who live at very high altitudes live significantly longer; they have a lower incidence of cancer (Weinberg, et al., 1987) and heart disease (Mortimer, et al., 1977), and other degenerative conditions, than people who live near sea level.

At high altitude CO_2 is in greater presence, and O_2 is in less. A Russian doctor named Konstantin Buteyko is most responsible for drawing attention to the importance of carbon dioxide for body metabolism and how the lack of it can cause chronic diseases. A molecule of carbon dioxide (CO_2)

consists of one carbon and two oxygen atoms. Colorless and odorless, it is hard to detect. The amount of carbon dioxide in the atmosphere has been in flux throughout the Earth's history.

The Importance of CO_2

Those who engaged in moderate to high-intensity exercise for at least 30 minutes a day were 50 percent less likely to develop cancer compared with the other men. Increased oxygen consumption associated with moderate to high-intensity exercise appears to reduce the risk of cancer, a new study has found. The Finnish study included 2,560 men, aged 42 to 61, whose leisure-time physical activity was assessed over one year. None of the men had a history of cancer, according to the report published online July 28 in the *British Journal of Sports Medicine*. The researchers found that an increase of 1.2 metabolic units (oxygen consumption) was related to a decreased risk of cancer death, especially in lung and gastrointestinal cancers, after they took into account factors such as age, smoking, alcohol consumption, body mass index, and fiber/fat intake.

Through the years I have laughed at the detractors of using sodium bicarbonate to treat cancer, knowing that they had not the slightest idea of what they are talking about. Medical Grade Carbon Dioxide USP is utilized in critical care areas of the hospital! The medical uses of carbon dioxide include the following, but be sure to add cancer and diabetes to the list:

- Inflation gas, for minimal invasive surgery (laparoscopy, endoscopy, arthroscopy), to enlarge and stabilize body cavities for better visibility of the surgical field.

- To increase the depth of respiration and help overcome breath holding and bronchial spasms during various procedures.

- To stimulate respiration for various reasons (i.e. chronic respiratory obstruction removal, hyperventilation).

- To increase cerebral blood flow during some surgeries.

- For clinical and physiological investigations.

Carbon dioxide gas protects against tissue damage in the operative field, in open-heart surgery. Carbon dioxide insufflation into the abdominal cavity results in the reduction of oxidative stress. Without CO_2 we would all die as well as everything else on earth. So why on earth would anyone want to tax a good thing?

CO_2 Field Flooding reduces oxidative stress in open-heart surgery. Dr. M. Persson and Dr. Van der Linden have demonstrated that carbon dioxide gas protects against tissue damage in the operative field by maintaining humidity and temperature in the open-heart surgery-related model environment. These scientists are saying that carbon dioxide insufflation into the abdominal cavity results in the reduction of oxidative stress.

Dr. Gerald Marsh tells us that five hundred million years ago, carbon dioxide concentrations were over 13 times current levels, and not until about 20 million years ago did carbon dioxide levels drop to a little less than twice what they are today.[2] Since 1750 the concentration in the air has risen from 278 parts per million (ppm) of CO_2 to more than 380 ppm, making it easier for plants to acquire the CO_2 needed for rapid growth. Scientists generally suggest that raised CO_2 levels will boost the yields of mainstream crops, such as maize, rice, and soy, by about 13 per cent.

The complicated world of oxygen, carbon dioxide, and tissue and tumor pH are important areas because our body simply cannot fight disease if its pH is not properly balanced. Consequently the oxygen-carrying capacity of our cells becomes compromised. It's really simple—higher pH conditions lead to higher O_2 levels, and in oxygen being delivered to where it is needed.

CO_2 Medicine

Carbon dioxide gas (CO_2) is generated and delivered to skin tissue, and it results in more oxygen release from blood vessels. It activates erythrocytes to supply more oxygen to dermal cells and therefore, activates cell metabolism. Natural biological functions of the skin can be maximized and all kinds of skin problems can be settled at cell level. CO_2 is a serious medicine. Not only is it used in emergency rooms, but also CO_2 is an essential food, not only for plants, but also for us. We simply do not work right when CO_2 and bicarbonate levels are low in the blood.

CO_2 Footbath Therapy

Carbon dioxide footbath therapy was developed as a means for healing diabetic foot and other ischemic ulcers. The only treatment that comes close to helping diabetes is magnesium therapy, which combines beautifully in baths with sodium bicarbonate and CO_2 medicine therapies.

Among the most severe complications associated with diabetes, mellitus are the deep tissue lesions of the foot known collectively as "diabetic foot." Until recently, the lack of an effective therapy for diabetic foot has led many patients with such complications down an inexorable and tragic path toward amputation of the foot. Oxygen delivered at higher concentrations gives the same effect. The secret to this is that oxygen and carbon dioxide are twin sisters or two sides of an interesting coin. Less oxygen is delivered in the face of carbon dioxide deficiencies, while healthy CO_2 levels insures plenty of oxygen gets delivered.

Bath Bombs

In addition to the carbon dioxide gel there are *Bath Bombs*, that can be added to a person's bath and can be crucial in helping a person recover from diseases including cancer. The same Japanese company that makes the gel for women makes a tablet that you put in the bath, and one soaks in the CO_2 right from the bath water. It is like loading up the tub with sodium bicarbonate, but in this case it is sodium bicarbonate mixed with citric acid, which breaks down the sodium bicarbonate into CO_2 micro bubbles, which is much more absorbable then sodium bicarbonate. CO_2 permeability through cell membrane is 25 times more than O_2.

The good news is that you can make *Bath Bombs* yourself or buy them with a variety of good smells for delicious medicinal baths. Treatment using natural carbon dioxide springs was common in Germany long before treatment with artificial CO_2—enriched water began in Japan. But if you go to any of the many *Bath Bomb* sites you will not find a word about the medical effects.

> *CO_2 water bathing helps reduce pulse and high blood pressure score, improves venous blood returning to the heart, and an increase of peripheral blood flow.*

Why does it Work?

Most of the CO_2 in the body is in the form of bicarbonate (HCO_3^-). Therefore, the CO_2 blood test is really a measure of your blood bicarbonate level. The normal range is 23 to 29 mEq/L (milliequivalent per liter).

> *If the level of carbon dioxide in the blood is lower than normal, then this leads to difficulties in releasing oxygen from hemoglobin.*

Some background medical information is quite revealing about the power *Bath Bombs* and sodium bicarbonate baths (as well as oral administration), as well as *rebreathing retraining,* all of which help restore blood CO_2/bicarbonate levels to normal.

Some of the diseases that are related to low CO_2 levels are:

- Addison disease
- Diarrhea
- Ethylene glycol poisoning
- Ketoacidosis
- Kidney disease

- Lactic acidosis
- Metabolic acidosis
- Methanol poisoning
- Salicylate toxicity (such as aspirin overdose)

The blood carries carbon dioxide to your lungs, where it is exhaled. More than 90 percent of carbon dioxide in your blood exists in the form of bicarbonate (HCO_3). The rest of the carbon dioxide is either dissolved carbon dioxide gas (CO_2) or carbonic acid ($H2CO_3$). Your kidneys and lungs balance the levels of carbon dioxide, bicarbonate, and carbonic acid in the blood.

Taking sodium bicarbonate orally or bathing in a tub saturated with it results in a shift of the body's pH to less acidic and more alkaline. That is because baking soda is an electron donor. As the pH rises, so does cellular voltage and cellular oxygen levels. These *Bath Bombs* or tablets take sodium bicarbonate medicine to another level by breaking down the sodium bicarbonate, with citric acid, to make CO_2 micro-bubbles. CO_2, which is only an alternative form of bicarbonate, is much more absorbable. Instead of loading up the bath with a kilo or two of bicarbonate, these tablets or *Bath Bombs* do the trick with just ounces of sodium bicarbonate.

We increase cell voltage, raise energy and performance levels of cellular activity, when we supplement with sodium bicarbonate, which has long been known as an excellent treatment for the kidneys—dialysis units use bicarbonate regularly.

Sodium bicarbonate + Citric Acid + Water = Radical chemical reaction produces CO_2 with lots of $-HCO_3$ and $+HCO_3$ with PH of 7.45.

pH Balance

Inflammation is inseparable from lower pH, oxygen, CO_2, and cell energy levels, which of course would track with cell temperature, respiration and elimination. A grand unification theory of medicine would describe this area of physiology where certain things are happening simultaneously with others. There is a point where one cannot separate out oxygen from CO_2

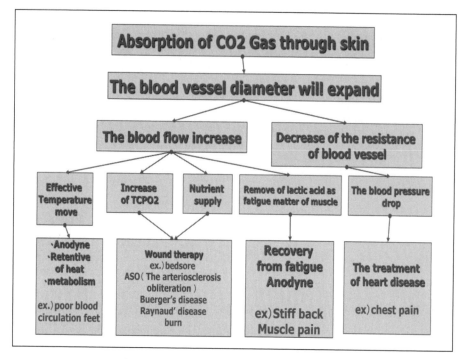

Figure 9.1   Flowchart of CO_2 Bathing Effect

levels because they are locked into a tight mathematical relationship with each other. The same is true about pH and cell voltage. As CO_2 levels go south with O_2 levels, pH dives as does cell voltage.

With inflammation, we also have viral, bacterial and fungal sharks ready to start biting on tissues until the entire process leads to degenerative diseases and cancer. Most infections do not take hold on strong healthy tissues. What is that level of life where we cannot break things apart without betraying their true nature? Is it that level where CO_2 levels bind tightly with O_2 levels? Is it the same place where pH and cell voltage track each other?

A grand unification theory of medicine would describe a certain point in physiology where certain things are happening simultaneously with others. There is a point where one cannot separate out oxygen from CO_2 levels because they are locked into a tight mathematical relationship with each other. Same is true about pH and cell voltage. As CO_2 levels go south with O_2 levels, pH dives as does cell voltage.

Imagine going into a cell and surrounding tissues in your mind and listen to the beautiful singing of healthy and happy cells, all of which are singing in healthy resonating frequencies and amplitudes of energy. But move past an area of inflammation and the sights and songs change.

The Key to Oxygen

The key to oxygen is not more oxygen, but more carbon dioxide, which is a nutritious gas, not a poison. Doctors at the Department of Anaesthesia and Medical-Surgical Intensive Care Unit, Toronto General Hospital in Ontario, Canada say that, "Accumulating clinical and basic scientific evidence points to an active role for carbon dioxide in organ injury, in which raised concentrations of carbon dioxide are protective and low concentrations are injurious."

Carbon dioxide executes uncountable functions in the human organism. Among them are: repair of alveoli in lungs, stability of the nerve cells, regulation of pulse, normal immunity, blood pressure maintenance, dilation of bronchi and bronchioles, regulation of blood pH, sleep control, relaxation of muscle cells, release of O_2 in capillaries (the Bohr effect), weight monitoring, and tens of other essential functions.

Hemoglobin helps to transport hydrogen ions and carbon dioxide in addition to transporting oxygen. However, transport by hemoglobin accounts for only about 14 percent of the total transport of these species; both hydrogen ions and carbon dioxide are also transported in the blood as bicarbonate (HCO_3^-), formed spontaneously or through the action of carbonic anhydrase.

In all serious disease states we find a concomitant low-oxygen state. Low oxygen in the body tissues is a sure indicator for disease. Hypoxia, or lack of oxygen in the tissues, is the fundamental cause for all degenerative disease.
—Dr. Stephen Levine Molecular Biologist

Sodium bicarbonate (baking soda) is the stunning medicine it is because it puts doctors' and patients' fingers on the CO_2 pulse of the body. Bicarbonate intake raises the CO_2 levels in the blood. On top of everything is the fact that CO_2 is a key regulator of inflammatory reactions due to control of cell's oxygen supply. *Bicarbonate also regulates inflammatory reactions with rapid changes in tissue and fluid pH.*

In order to survive, the body must maintain proper acid/alkaline (pH) balance because when it does not do so, tissue oxygen levels suffer. The optimum (and required) pH of the blood is somewhat alkaline, between

7.35 and 7.45. *Only in this range is the blood richly supplied with oxygen.* (Realize that if your blood pH varies just a little bit, it can kill you.) The vast majority of terminal cancer patients are more acidic than normal healthy people, meaning their tissues have a very low pH and very low levels of oxygen throughout their entire body.

Oxygen, Inflammation and Hypoxia-Inducible Factor (HIF-1)

Scientists in Germany have shown that the microenvironment of inflamed and injured tissues are typically characterized by low levels of oxygen and glucose and high levels of inflammatory cytokines, reactive oxygen, nitrogen species, and metabolites. Recent medical research has suggested that there is a strong link between cell hypoxia (oxygen deficiency in cells) and chronic inflammatory processes.

Inflammation is the most common causes of tissue hypoxia and/or decreased circulation. Both inflamed tissues, as well as the areas surrounding malignant tumors, are characterized by hypoxia and low concentrations of glucose. Inflammation can lead to sepsis, circulatory collapse, and ultimately multi-system organ failure.

Tissue hypoxia is manifested in increased levels of hypoxia-inducible factor (HIF-1) (this factor and cell hypoxia are key factors in the progress of cancer). Elevated HIF-1 triggers a cascade of events with involvement of pro-inflammatory transcription factors such as nuclear factor kappa B (or NF-kappa B) and activator protein AP-1.

Researchers have found that low levels of magnesium suppresses reactive-oxygen-species- (ROS) induced HIF-1. When oxygen levels fall, things get dangerous on a cell level because at low levels gene expression changes. HIF-1a regulates the expression of at least 30 genes when oxygen levels are low. Magnesium deficiency depresses HIF-1a activity.

This is all-important because it is often an excessive inflammatory immune response (sepsis) that contributes to the patient's death. On intensive care units, *sepsis is the second-most common cause of death worldwide.* Patients with a severely compromised immune system face attack from Candida fungal infections, which become life threatening because of the high risk of sepsis.

Doctors who make fun of Dr. Tullio Simonini's theories about cancer being a fungus should look at themselves in the mirror and look at some medical facts that do suggest that at a minimum late stage cancer patients are suffering from immune exhaustion and overgrowth of Candida and other pathogens. We will spend quite some time later in this book delving into this most interesting issue.

Cancer and HIF-1

"Radiation and chemotherapy do kill most solid tumor cells, but in the cells that survive, the therapies drive an increase in HIF-1, which cells use to get the oxygen they need by increasing blood vessel growth into the tumor. Solid tumors generally have low supplies of oxygen, and HIF-1 helps them get the oxygen they need," explains Dr. Mark W. Dewhirst, professor of radiation oncology at Duke University Medical Center.

Dr. Holger K. Eltzschig, a professor of anesthesiology, medicine, cell biology, and immunology at the University of Colorado School of Medicine, says, "Understanding how hypoxia is linked to inflammation may help save lives. By focusing on the molecular pathways the body uses to battle hypoxia, we may be able help patients who undergo organ transplants, who suffer from infections, or who have cancer."

Researchers found that an increase of 1.2 metabolic units (oxygen consumption) was related to a decreased risk of cancer death, especially in lung and gastrointestinal cancers.[3] In order for cancer to "establish" a foothold in the body, it has to be deprived of oxygen and become acidic. Drs. D. F. Treacher and R. M. Leach write, "Prevention, early identification, and correction of tissue hypoxia are essential skills. If oxygen supply fails, even for a few minutes, tissue hypoxaemia may develop resulting in anaerobic metabolism and production of lactate."[4] Anything that threatens the oxygen-carrying capacity of the human body will promote cancer growth. Likewise any therapy that improves the oxygen function can be expected to enhance the body's defenses against cancer.

The Key Drivers of Cancer Growth—Scientific Findings

Scientists have recently confirmed, yet again, that long-term lack of oxygen in cells is the key driver of cancer growth. Who says so now? Dr. Ying Xu, Regents-Georgia Research Alliance Eminent Scholar and professor of bioinformatics and computational biology in the Franklin College of Arts and Sciences. His study was published in the *Journal of Molecular Cell Biology* in 2012. "Cancer drugs try to get to the root—at the molecular level—of a particular mutation, but the cancer often bypasses it," Xu said. "So we think that possibly genetic mutations may not be the main driver of cancer."[5]

Every doctor learned back in medical school all about Dr. Otto Warburg's discovery in the 1930s, when he discovered the main biochemical cause of cancer or what differentiates a cancer cell from a normal, healthy cell. Dr. Warburg was awarded the Nobel Prize for his important work. Dr. Warburg said, "Cancer, above all other diseases, has countless secondary causes.

Almost anything can cause cancer. But, even for cancer, there is only one prime cause. The prime cause of cancer is the replacement of the respiration of oxygen (oxidation of sugar) in normal body cells by fermentation of sugar. In every case, during the cancer development, the oxygen respiration always falls, fermentation appears, and the highly differentiated cells are transformed into fermenting anaerobes, which have lost all their body functions and retain only the now useless property of growth and replication."

Cancer has a primary characteristic by which it can be measured. "It is the replacement of normal oxygen respiration of the body's cells by an anaerobic [for example, oxygen-deficient] cell respiration," said Warburg. This tells us that cancer metabolizes much differently than normal cells. Normal cells need oxygen. Cancer cells despise oxygen. Another thing this tells us is that cancer metabolizes through a process of fermentation. The metabolism of cancer is approximately eight times greater than the metabolism of normal cells (that's why they love sugar so much), but Warburg forgot to tell the world—not only are the oxygen levels low, but so are carbon dioxide (CO_2) levels. And he did not tell a soul that by breathing too fast (as most people do) they are getting rid of too much CO_2, and that is what is driving down the oxygen levels to the point that cells turn cancerous.

Otto Warburg was telling us that the cellular metabolism of cancer cells matches closely those of yeast or mold or fungus—that is, the cells ferment sugar/glucose/dextrose rather than oxidize it via the cellular mitochondria. So it follows logically that the same medical approach that successfully targets cancer would do the same for these yeasts, molds, and fungus. Warburg had only part of the story, and no one has put the finishing chapter in so we can finally come to rest with a full understanding and appreciation of what we are facing when cancer knocks on our door. Natural Allopathic Medicine approaches the core problem of oxygen from many directions at once.

Dr. Lesley Walker, Cancer Research UK's director of cancer information, said, "For a long time scientists have been looking for ways to boost the oxygen supply to tumors to improve response to treatment." He was referring to treatment with radiation, but this would apply very much to a whole range of natural treatments.

Oncologists are baffled by the unpredictability of cancers cells. Even after "seemingly" effective treatments, crafty cancer cells are able to hide out in patients and then resurface later on. It's known that low oxygen levels in tumors can be used to predict cancer recurrence in men with intermediate-risk prostate cancer even before they receive radiation therapy.

"We've not only shown that men do worse if they have low oxygen levels (hypoxia) in their prostate cancer, but that they also do worse over a shorter period of time," says Dr. Michael Milosevic, radiation oncologist in the PMH Cancer Program, UHN. "These patients seem to develop cancer recurrence within only a few years of completing treatment." Dr. Milosevic and colleagues measured oxygen levels in 247 men with localized prostate cancer prior to radiation therapy and followed them for a median of 6.6 years. Low oxygen in the tumors predicted early relapse after radiation treatment. It was also the *only* identified factor that predicted local recurrence during follow-up.[6]

Dr. Rockwell from Yale University School of Medicine (USA) studied malignant changes on the cellular level and wrote, "The physiological effects of hypoxia and the associated micro environmental inadequacies increase mutation rates, select for cells deficient in normal pathways of programmed cell death, and contribute to the development of an increasingly invasive, metastatic phenotype"[7]

Professor Gillies McKenna, director of the UK-MRC Gray Institute for Radiation Oncology & Biology, said, "We are very excited to have uncovered this brand new approach to cancer treatment where the drugs prime the cancer cells for radiotherapy. You might expect that by increasing an oxygen supply to tumor cells, you would help them grow. But actually by oxygenating the cell with a better blood supply, we enable radiotherapy and chemotherapy to do a better job of killing them." The research was published in the journal *Cancer Today*, and again we see that oxygen therapy increases one's chances of winning the war on cancer.

Many studies have measured the link between oxygen partial pressure in cells (or expression of hypoxia inducible factors, their concentrations) and appearance, growth, and metastasis of tumors.[8,9,10] Sodium bicarbonate acts much like a bunker buster bomb—it blasts cancer with shock waves of oxygen and CO_2, thereby increasing cell voltage and raising pH into the alkaline range without harming the host.

Hypocapnia (lowered CO_2) leads to reduced oxygenation of all vital organs and tissues due to fast superficial breathing, vasoconstriction, and the suppressed Bohr effect. The Bohr effect explains oxygen release in capillaries or why red blood cells unload oxygen in tissues. The Bohr effect was first described in 1904 by the Danish physiologist Christian Bohr (father of famous physicist Niels Bohr). Christian Bohr stated that *at lower pH (more acidic environment, for example in tissues), hemoglobin will bind to oxygen with less affinity*. Since carbon dioxide is in direct equilibrium with the concentration of protons in the blood, increasing blood carbon dioxide content causes a decrease in acid pH, which leads to a decrease in affinity for oxygen by hemoglobin. This is exactly how sodium bicarbonate works. It increases CO_2 levels in the blood.

Injecting oxygen into cancerous tumors significantly boosts the chances of recovery, scientists at Oxford University say. They found that increasing the supply of O_2 strengthened blood vessels in cancer cells, making chemotherapy more effective. In a series of experiments on mice, *cells that were damaged and weak had a constricted oxygen supply* and were less sensitive to radiotherapy treatments.

Basic scientific research confirms the benefits of using sodium bicarbonate in cancer treatment. Dr. Julian Whitaker and Mark McCarty write, "The degree to which pH is depressed in tumors—as mirrored by their lactate levels—tends to correlate with prognosis, the more acidic tumors being associated with poorer outcome. In part, this phenomenon may reflect the fact that tumor acidity is serving as a marker for HIF-1 activation, which works in a variety of complementary ways to boost tumor capacity for invasion, metastasis, angiogenesis, and chemoresistance. However, there is increasing evidence that extracellular acidity *per se* contributes to the aggressiveness of cancer cells, boosting extracellular proteolytic activities, expression of pro-angiogenic factors, and metastatic capacity."

Researchers have investigated the very reasonable assumption that increased systemic concentrations of pH buffers would lead to reduced intratumoral and peritumoral acidosis and, as a result, would inhibit malignant growth. It has been shown that increased serum concentrations of the sodium bicarbonate ($NaHCO_3$) can be achieved via oral intake.[11] Researchers found that consequent reduction of tumor acid concentrations significantly reduces tumor growth and invasion.[12]

Oral $NaHCO_3$ selectively increased the pH of tumors and reduced the formation of spontaneous metastases in mouse models of metastatic breast cancer. $NaHCO_3$ therapy also reduced the rate of lymph node involvement and significantly reduced the formation of hepatic metastases. Acid pH was shown to increase the release of active cathepsin B, an important matrix remodeling protease.[13] Magnetic resonance spectroscopy (MRS) has shown that the pH of MCF-7 human breast cancer xenografts can be effectively and significantly raised with sodium bicarbonate in drinking water.[14]

10. Carbon Dioxide

Public opinion tends to think of carbon dioxide as a waste product or even a poison. (It is sometimes confused with carbon monoxide, which is a poison). Waste means toxic, but everything is toxic, including water, in the allopathic paradigm where the dose makes the poison. CO_2 is a waste product that we need. It is essential for life. It comes from living life, and it goes back into creating life. Carbon dioxide gas makes plants grow. It is a life gas not a death gas. You can treat cancer with it because increased systemic concentrations of pH buffers leads to reduced intratumoral and peritumoral acidosis and, as a result, inhibit malignant growth of cancer.

A UN panel of climate scientists recently found with 95 percent certainty that humans are responsible for the earth's warming temperatures, up from 90 percent certainty six years ago. They concluded that only a rapid reduction in greenhouse gas emissions could possibly reverse the global warming trend. Notice these people are in doubt. Forget what the actual numbers are because they vary from computer to computer depending on what kind of assumptions scientists are making. NASA says that carbon dioxide is actually having a cooling effect in the upper atmosphere and on earth.

Carbon Dioxide Deficiency

Little does anyone know, that a lack of carbon dioxide is harmful, and even less understand that carbon dioxide is as fundamental a component of living matter as oxygen. If a carbon dioxide deficiency continues for a long time then it can be responsible for diseases, aging and even cancer. The ancient forms of medicine knew that for increased vitality and freedom from disease, good habits of breathing must be formed. They knew that poor breathing reduces our vitality and opens the door to disease.

The principle role of breathing is, of course, to stay alive! One of the ways in which breathing does this is through seeking to maintain an optimum internal oxygen-carbon dioxide balance. The important thing is not how much oxygen or how much carbon dioxide you have in your system, but rather the relationship between the two gases—between carbon dioxide and oxygen. Too much oxygen (relative to the level of carbon dioxide) and we feel agitated and jumpy. Too much carbon dioxide (again, relative to the level of oxygen) and we feel sluggish and sleepy and tired.

Poor oxygenation or hypoxia appears to be a favorable environment for cancer development, whereas good oxygenation favors healthy tissue growth. Increasing CO_2 levels through the use of sodium bicarbonate is good in cancer treatment because bicarbonate drives up CO_2 levels in the blood, which increases oxygenation to the cells.

The best way to produce carbon dioxide is from physical activity, but most people with chronic illness and cancer unfortunately do not exercise. Understanding how important bicarbonate and CO_2 physiology can be to the chronically ill person involves understanding the basic physiology of carbon dioxide. Yes, women can make themselves more beautiful with CO_2 masks, but we can make patients more beautiful and a lot more comfortable when we resolve their bedsores, gangrene, eczema, and fatigue with CO_2. Physical activity and sports is good for us because it raises CO_2 concentrations though there are limits to everything including a good thing like CO_2. Therefore, we do have, as we do for magnesium and everything else, a way of blowing off excess.

Oxygen and Carbon Dioxide Dependency

"Another natural misconception is that oxygen and carbon dioxide are so far antagonistic that a gain of one in the blood necessarily involves a corresponding loss of the other. On the contrary, although each tends to raise the pressure and thus promote the diffusion of the other, the two gases are held and transported in the blood by different means; oxygen is carried by the hemoglobin in the corpuscles, while carbon dioxide is combined with alkali in the plasma. A sample of blood may be high in both gases or low in both gases. Under clinical conditions, low oxygen and low carbon dioxide generally occur together. Therapeutic increase of carbon dioxide, by inhalation of this gas diluted in air, is often an effective means of improving the oxygenation of the blood and tissues."[1]

Few people know that a decreased level of carbon dioxide in the blood leads to decreased oxygen supply to the cells in the body including in the brain, heart, and kidneys. Carbon dioxide (CO_2) was found at the end of the

19th century by scientists Bohr and Verigo to be responsible for the bond between oxygen and hemoglobin. If the level of carbon dioxide in the blood is lower than normal, then this leads to difficulties in releasing oxygen from hemoglobin. Hence, the Verigo-Bohr law—according to the Verigo-Bohr effect, we can state that a CO_2 deficit caused by deep breathing leads to oxygen starvation in the cells of the body.

Scientific Findings

Way back in the 19th century, Zuntz, in Berlin, recognized that carbon dioxide, unlike oxygen, is not carried by hemoglobin. He showed that in the blood, carbon dioxide is combined with bases, chiefly as sodium bicarbonate, which plays a part in acid-alkaline balance. Most of the carbon dioxide is dissolved in the plasma, both in simple solution and that combined with alkali into the bicarbonates.

According to the Verigo-Bohr effect (which we will look at below), we can state that a CO_2 deficit caused by deep breathing leads to oxygen starvation in the cells of the body. This state is known as hypoxia, and it badly affects the nervous system. Chronic hidden hyperventilation (over-breathing) is very common amongst western populations, leading to impaired oxygenation of body tissues. But what is actually driving down the O_2 levels is the hyperventilation. It's getting rid of too much CO_2. Meaning we need the CO_2 almost as much as we need the O_2 because, as we shall also see below, the two are married to each other in an eternal physiology dance.

Most people have unhealthy breathing habits. They hold their breath or breathe high in the chest or in a shallow, irregular manner. These patterns have been unconsciously adopted, accidentally formed, or emotionally impressed. Certain "typical" breathing patterns actually trigger physiological and psychological stress, and anxiety reactions. Babies know how to breathe, and you can see their belly expand as the diaphragm moved down. Adults breathe more through expanding their chest cavity, and it takes training and discipline to return to more natural breathing patterns.

Biologist Dr. Ray Peat tells us that "breathing pure oxygen lowers the oxygen content of tissues; breathing rarefied air, or air with carbon dioxide, oxygenates and energizes the tissues; if this seems upside down, it's because medical physiology has been taught upside down. And respiratory physiology holds the key to the special functions of all the organs and too many of their basic pathological changes." [2] People who live at very high altitudes live significantly longer; they have a lower incidence of cancer (Weinberg, et al., 1987) and heart disease (Mortimer, et al., 1977), and other degenerative conditions, than people who live near sea level.

Dr. Peat continues saying that, "Breathing too much oxygen displaces too much carbon dioxide, provoking an increase in lactic acid; too much lactate displaces both oxygen and carbon dioxide. Lactate itself tends to suppress respiration. Oxygen toxicity and hyperventilation create a systemic deficiency of carbon dioxide. It is this carbon dioxide deficiency that makes breathing more difficult in pure oxygen, that impairs the heart's ability to work, and that increases the resistance of blood vessels, impairing circulation and oxygen delivery to tissues. In conditions that permit greater carbon dioxide retention, circulation is improved and the heart works more effectively. Carbon dioxide inhibits the production of lactic acid, and lactic acid lowers carbon dioxide's concentration in a variety of ways."

The presence of lactic acid, which indicates stress or defective respiration, interferes with energy metabolism in ways that tend to be self-promoting. Harry Rubin's experiments demonstrated that cells become cancerous before genetic changes appear. The mere presence of lactic acid can make cells more susceptible to the transformation into cancer cells. (Mothersill, et al.,1983.) The implications of this for the increased susceptibility to cancer during long term stress are obvious.

"Otto Warburg established that lactic acid production is a fundamental property of cancer. It is, to a great degree, the lactic acid which triggers the defensive reactions of the organism, leading to tissue wasting from excessive glucocorticoid hormone," says Dr. Peat. Tumors do tend to be efficient at exporting lactate which drops the pH in the milieu of the tumor. The breakdown of glucose or glycogen produces lactate and hydrogen ions—for each lactate molecule, one hydrogen ion is formed.

It is carbon dioxide deficiency that impairs circulation and oxygen delivery to tissues. Carbon dioxide inhibits the production of lactic acid, and lactic acid lowers carbon dioxide's concentration in a variety of ways.
—Dr. Ray Peat

Thus, we can begin to see that it is the lack of carbon dioxide in the body which is a cause of many disturbances in the metabolism of cells and tissues, which, in turn, can lead to disease. Dr. Buteyko said, "CO_2 is the main source of nutrition for any living matter on Earth. Plants obtain CO_2 from the air and provide the main source of nourishment for animals, while both plants and animals are nourishment for us. The great resource of CO_2 in the air was formed in pre-historical times when the amount was about 10 percent."

Increasing Carbon Dioxide

The best way to produce carbon dioxide is from physical activity but most people with chronic illness and cancer unfortunately do not exercise. Understanding how important sodium bicarbonate can be to the chronically ill person involves understanding the basic physiology of carbon dioxide. This leads us directly to our breath, and we must understand and take conscious control of it, so we optimize our breathing and CO_2 and thus, oxygen levels. Over breathing really is a kind of self-suffocation, when taken to the extreme, because we are driving down CO_2 levels and that actually decreases oxygen to the cells.

There are different techniques designed for increasing carbon dioxide levels in the blood. Dr. Buteyko developed a system where by breathing techniques controlled asthma. The ancient yogis with their yogic breathing, and NASA controls spaceship climates with these issues in mind. Natural medicine makes proper breathing important because the central mechanism to maintain CO_2 levels is correct breathing.[3] The clinical choice often is IV injection of bicarbonate in emergency situations, but the rest of us can take the easy inexpensive way using oral sodium bicarbonate.

About 80 percent of the CO_2 formed by metabolism is transported from tissues to lungs as bicarbonate ions dissolved in the water phases of red cells and plasma. The catalyzed hydration of CO_2 to bicarbonate takes place in the erythrocytes, but most of the bicarbonate thus formed must be exchanged with extracellular chloride to make full use of the carbon dioxide transporting capacity of the blood. This is an important reason why magnesium chloride is not only the ideal form of magnesium, but also the reason to combine magnesium chloride with bicarbonate. Chloride is another basic substance that runs parallel biological processes.

The anion transport capacity of the red cell membrane is among the largest ionic transport capacities of any biological membrane. Exchange diffusion of chloride and bicarbonate is nevertheless a rate-limiting step for the transfer of CO_2 from tissues to lungs.[4] Baking soda (sodium bicarbonate) immediately reacts when it mixes with stomach acid. $NaHCO_3 + HCl \rightarrow NaCl + H_2O + CO_2$. That is: Sodium bicarbonate + stomach acid yields salt + water + carbon dioxide. This is the physiological reason why bicarbonate is such an effective medicine; it instantly offers a return to more normal CO_2 levels which drives more oxygen into the tissues. This is not something cancer cells enjoy.

So now that we know something about carbon dioxide it's not something we need to be afraid of, and certainly we don't want anyone putting a tax on it, for the trees, at least, are loving that there is more of it in the air.

If there is any truth in the fact that more CO_2 in the air has a warming affect, then perhaps in the end, we will be thankful when it gets really cold that it is not as cold as it might be if we had not filled the air with so much of it due to human activity.

Carbonic Acid

CO_2 is a gas at room temperature, and consists of a central carbon atom and two oxygen atoms arranged in a linear fashion. When dissolved into water, the CO_2 becomes hydrated to form carbonic acid (H_2CO_3). This hydration step takes a few seconds, though that may seem fast, many organisms from bacteria to humans use an enzyme called carbonic anhydrase to greatly speed up the process.

Once carbonic acid forms, it very quickly equilibrates with the other acids and bases in solution. It can, for example, lose one or two protons (H+). The extent to which this happens depends upon the pH and a variety of other factors. In seawater at pH 8.1, most of it (87 percent) will lose one proton to form bicarbonate, a small amount will lose two protons to form carbonate (13 percent), and a very small amount will remain as H_2CO_3 (1 percent). All of these forms, however, interconvert faster than the blink of an eye, so one cannot identify one as carbonate and one as bicarbonate for more than a tiny fraction of a second. All one can really say is that on average X percent is in the form of bicarbonate, and Y percent in the form of carbonate.[5] Total CO_2 is defined as the sum of carbonic acid and bicarbonate.

Carbonic acid plays a very important role as a buffer in our blood. The equilibrium between carbon dioxide and carbonic acid is very important for controlling the acidity of body fluids, and the carbonic anhydrase increases the reaction rate by a factor of nearly a billion to keep the fluids at a stable pH. Carbon dioxide does change the pH of water. This is how it works:

Carbon dioxide dissolves slightly in water to form a weak acid called carbonic acid, H_2CO_3, according to the following reaction:

$$CO_2 + H_2O \rightarrow H_2CO_3$$

After that, carbonic acid reacts slightly and reversibly in water to form a hydronium cation, H3O+, and the bicarbonate ion, HCO_3^-, according to the following reaction:

$$H_2CO_3 + H_2O \rightarrow HCO_3^- + H_3O^+$$

In the basement of human physiology are these lightning fast translations, so for all intent and purpose, drinking sparkling water is very similar to drinking bicarbonate water. And in fact, we can add sodium bicarbonate to the sparkling water we can easily and joyfully make at home. Scientists have found out in animal studies that sparkling water stimulates HCO_3^- secretion in both the stomach and the duodenum[6], but I am not sure whether it is actually being secreted or just transformed. The point is clear though that CO_2 and HCO_3^- (bicarbonate ions) are closely related and are interchangeable in the presence of water.

The normal ratio of bicarbonate to carbonic acid at normal pH is around 20:1; total CO_2 will therefore be about 5 percent higher than serum bicarbonate. When you observe a difference between total CO_2 and bicarbonate that is larger than 5 percent, the patient will be acidic. In aqueous solution, carbonic acid dissociates into a bicarbonate ion and a proton or into carbon dioxide and water depending on the conditions such as pH and the relative concentrations of each of the products, for example carbon dioxide and bicarbonate.

The carbonic acid, carbon dioxide bicarbonate axis represents the main buffers against dangerous pH changes; a buffer is a substance that resists changes in pH (acid concentration) by undergoing a reversible reaction. When weak acids are added to a buffer solution, the resulting change in pH is less than it would have been if the buffer were not present. When hydrogen ion (H+) is added, much of the hydrogen is taken up by the salt of the buffering acid. With bicarbonate, H^+ bonds to HCO_3^- to form H_2CO_3, which is a weak acid. The main characteristic of a buffer is that the reaction is reversible—the hydrogen ion can be given back.

Staying Safely Hydrated

If all the above is confusing, it's understandable unless you have a background in chemistry. What is vital to know and understand is that raising the pH increases oxygen binding to hemoglobin, allowing more total oxygen to be carried. Drinking alkaline water, ingesting sodium bicarbonate, and even drinking sparkling water, especially if it contains high bicarbonate levels, will alkalinize the blood and increase oxygen delivery to the cells.

The perfect water would be rich in *magnesium* (magnesium also increases O_2 carrying capacity) and calcium and low in sodium chloride," says Roberta Anding, director of sports nutrition at the Texas Medical Center, and a dietitian for the Houston Texans football team. According to a study in the *American Journal of Medicine,* that means more than 48 milligrams of magnesium and 85 milligrams of calcium per liter, and fewer than 195 milligrams of sodium per liter. Just because water has bubbles, either because they've been forced in by the manufacturer, by you at home, or because they occurred naturally from a spring, doesn't mean it also contains more or less of certain minerals than still water.

Diabetics and everyone else need to make a conscious effort to keep fully hydrated. Lack of water can lead to dehydration, a condition that occurs when you don't have enough water in your body to carry on normal functions. Even mild dehydration—as little as a 1 percent to 2 percent loss of your body weight—can sap your energy and make you tired. Dehydration poses a particular health risk for the very young and the very old.

Substitute sparkling water for alcoholic drinks, coffee and colas, all of which are acidic and dehydrating, is a pleasurable way of increasing hydration. Water is the most basic of all medicines, and it is possible to make increased water intake pleasurable and highly medicinal.

11. The pH Story—
Acid Death Vs Alkaline Life

Proteins can be modified both in vivo and in vitro by increases in acidity. In fact pH is the regulatory authority that controls most cellular processes. The pH balance of the human bloodstream is recognized by medical physiology texts as one of the most important biochemical balances in all of human body chemistry. As mentioned previously, pH is the acronym for "Potential Hydrogen". In definition, it is the degree of concentration of hydrogen ions in a substance or solution. It is measured on a logarithmic scale from 0 to 14. Higher numbers mean a substance is more alkaline in nature and there is a greater potential for absorbing more hydrogen ions. Lower numbers indicate more acidity with less potential for absorbing hydrogen ions.

> *The extracellular (interstitial) pH (pHe) of solid tumours is significantly more acidic compared to normal tissues.* [1]

Our body pH is very important because pH controls the speed of our body's biochemical reactions. It does this by controlling the speed of enzyme activity, as well as the speed that electricity moves through our body. The higher (more alkaline) the pH of a substance or solution, the more electrical resistance that substance or solution holds. Therefore, electricity travels slower with higher pH. If we say something has an acid pH, we are saying it is *hot and fast*. Alkaline pHon the other hand, bio-chemically speaking, is *slow and cool*. The closer the pH is to 7.35—7.45, the higher our level of health and well-being, and our ability to resist states of disease.

Body pH level changes have a profound effect on total body physiology.

Oxidative stress, which correlates directly with pH changes into the acidic, is especially dangerous to the mitochondria, which suffer the greatest under oxidative duress. Only by eliminating acid waste, restoring your body's pH balance, and preventing further accumulation of acid will we be able to lower our risk of cancer and other serious chronic diseases.

Dangers of an Acid pH

When we consume food that are high in acid or heavily processed, or food that causes an allergic response in our digestive systems, the food will not be absorbed properly into our bodies as nutrients. Instead, some of the food will be absorbed into the bloodstream as acid waste. The remainder of undigested food will linger in your intestines and putrefy, causing further release of acid into your bloodstream. The result is a general degeneration which creates the condition for cancer or its reoccurrence. This is a great problem with autistic children who suffer from what is called "leaky gut syndrome."

Improper digestion creates the perfect environment for bacteria and fungus to thrive. Where pathogens accumulate, inflammation follows. A reduction in body acid is possible through proper diet and supplements. Acidic blood pH levels, which cause toxic acid wastes (acidosis), is mostly unknown (outside of the emergency room), but is a dangerously destructive circumstance because it leads to cancer and other chronic diseases. When you have an acidic pH, your body is being silently burned down day-by-day. However, when you maintain an alkaline pH on a daily basis, your body can rebuild, repair, rejuvenate, and remain young. Yes, long term aging is very much related to pH permanently shifted toward the acidic. Our body's pH level regulates breathing, circulation, digestion, elimination, hormone production, and immune defense.

The first major line of defense against sickness, disease, and aging is the pH of your blood, and we can push this quite quickly into higher pH levels with sodium bicarbonate. This is why we can use bicarbonate in many clinical situations, even with the flu, for it will push the immune system through higher alkalinity into overdrive. The body prefers a slightly alkaline pH of approximately 7.4 in the blood and cells and if it drops below this for any length of time, it will suffer from the onset of degenerative disease or even acute infectious diseases like the flu. As our bodies becomes acidic, our body's oxygen level begins to drop, leaving us tired and fatigued, and this is what allows fungus, mold, parasites, bad bacteria, and viral infections to flourish and gain a hold throughout the body. When we become acidic we also start losing calcium out of the blood, the bones, as well as magnesium. Minerals are harnessed in a mandatory need to keep the blood pH slightly alkaline, but this becomes a losing game, for most people are also deficient in magnesium and other basic buffering minerals.

The great advantage of knowing the prime cause of a disease is that it can then be attacked logically and over a broad front.
—Dr. Otto Warburg

Dr. Otto Warburg, two times Nobel Prize winner, stated in his book *The Metabolism of Tumors* that the primary cause of cancer was the replacement of oxygen in the respiratory cell chemistry by the fermentation of sugar. The growth of cancer cells is initiated by a fermentation process, which can be triggered only in the absence of oxygen at the cell level. What Warburg was describing was a classic picture of acidic conditions. Just like overworked muscle cells manufacture lactic acid by-products as waste, cancerous cells spill lactic acid and other acidic compounds causing acid pH.

Patients receiving sodium bicarbonate achieved urine pHs of 6.5 as opposed to 5.6 with those receiving sodium chloride. This alkalinization is theorized to have a protective effect against the formation of free-radicals that may cause nephropathy.[2]
—Dr. Michael Metro

At a pH slightly above 7.4 cancer cells become dormant, and at pH 8.0 cancer cells will die while healthy cells will live. This has given rise to a variety of treatments based on increasing the alkalinity of the tissues such as vegetarian diet, raw foods, the drinking of fresh fruit, and vegetable juices, and dietary supplementation with alkaline minerals such as calcium, potassium, magnesium, cesium, and rubidium. But nothing can compare to the relatively instant alkalinizing power of sodium bicarbonate for safe and effective treatment of cancer. Cancer seems to grow slowly in a high acid environment (the acids cause it to partially destroy itself) and may actually grow more quickly as your body becomes more alkaline prior to reaching the healthy pH; which means reaching slightly above 7.4 where the cancer becomes dormant. Therefore, it is important to get the pH above 7.4 quickly and then to get the urinary pH up to 8.0.

Arthur C. Guyton, M.D., who is considered the world's most recognized author on human physiology, has spent the better part of his life studying the pH or acid/alkaline balance of the body. In his *Textbook of Medical Physiology* which is used to train medical students, he states, "The first step in maintaining health is to alkalize the body. The second step is to increase the number of negative hydrogen ions. These are the two most important aspects of homeostasis."

When a person's body becomes acidic they start to get a condition called *Blood Rouleau*. This condition is when the red blood cells stack up like pennies in a coin roll. The red blood cells are responsible for transporting oxygen and nutrients to the body and removing waste. When stacked up, the red blood cells cannot transport as much oxygen and nutrients to the body. Waste removal is also reduced because of lack of surface area on the red blood cells. A person in this condition often feels tired and tends to over eat because their body is starving. More protein and carbohydrates are consumed which leads to more *Blood Rouleau* due to the fact most carbohydrates and proteins are acidic. In this condition the white blood cells tend to be smaller and less active, which allows people to get sick easier due to less responsive immune system.

Oxygen cannot stick to blood cells if the pH of the blood is too acidic. You can breathe pure oxygen, but if the blood pH is acidic, the oxygen will not be able to be picked up by the blood cells. It is chemically impossible. The blood must be normal, and normal blood has a pH of around 7.4 pH. Any vestigial traces of oxygen that the acid-drenched blood cells manage to pick up are stripped off early. They are stripped off by the oxygen-starved cells along the way and never reach the deeper parts of the body where oxygen is most needed. Because the pH is acidic, carbon dioxide also is not transported efficiently and so builds up within the tissues leading both to cell death.

The strong acids in our bodies are those that are formed by the degradation of protein. These are sulfuric acid, phosphoric acid, and nitric acid. These are strong, like the battery acid in your car. Strong acids are strong in contradistinction to weak acids, such as vinegar and citrus juices. Weak acids do not ionize (break apart completely) when in solution; whereas, strong acids do.

Control of pH is crucial to neuronal function, given the high metabolic rates of acid production and sensitivity of electrical flow to changes of pH.

One of the main reasons we become acidic is from over-consumption of protein. Eating meat and dairy products may increase the risk of prostate cancer, research suggests.[3] Conversely mineral deficiencies are another reason, and when you combine high protein intake with decreasing intake of minerals you have a medical disaster in the making through lowering of pH. When protein breaks down in our bodies, they break into the above mentioned strong acids. These three acids must be excreted by the kidneys because they contain sulfur, phosphorus, or nitrogen, which cannot break down into water and carbon dioxide to be eliminated as the weak acids are. In their passage through the kidneys, these strong acids must take a basic mineral with them because in this way they are converted into their neutral salts and don't burn the kidneys on their way out. This would happen if these acids were excreted in their free acid form. The following information is from my still to be published book *Natural Allopathic Medicine*.

Few people are conscious of the decreasing value of vitamins, minerals, and proteins in the food we all eat. Our children are being caught between a hammer and a hard place. On one side they are being poisoned, and on the other they are being deprived of the very nutrition necessary to resist all the different toxicities that confronts them. Then, on top of everything else, our children's systems have to navigate through further deficiencies brought on by antibiotics that are used too often.

Intensive care medicine is the only place in regular medicine that pH is taken seriously. Arterial blood pH is measured frequently in intensive care because here the pH of the blood itself does change. Acidosis is a very serious condition that demands an immediate response in intensive care land; the response of choice of course is sodium bicarbonate. This book is about chronic acidosis, as well as treating cancerous tumors through a generalized manipulation of full body pH from acid to alkaline.

Changing the pH from Acid to Alkaline

Acid conditions alter virtually all cell and body functions and are considered to contribute in a fundamental sense to rapid aging and disease. The neutralization of damaging acid conditions in the body by carbonate sediments and bicarbonate solutions may be one of the main reasons that many animals and people live longer and stay healthier. Next time you hear a doctor or anyone else opposing or negating the importance of pH in health or disease, offer them a bottle of acid to drink or a coke. Both will make a point.

The oceans of the world are alkaline and contain carbonate sediments, bicarbonate ions, and relatively high concentrations of calcium and magnesium ions. We also know that the blood is also alkaline and is very similar in composition and properties to ocean water. That is why Navy doctors in WWII were able to substitute clean seawater for blood serum when they ran out of their medical supplies. People in the world who drink from natural water sources containing carbonate sediments, bicarbonate ions, and relatively high levels of mineral ions have superior health and longevity. The National Academy of Sciences and the associated National Research Council have evidence that groups of people demonstrate increased longevity and health if they reside in areas of the United States that have relatively high levels of bicarbonate ions and mineral ions in the drinking water. Numerous other expert studies around the world have found that people demonstrate increased longevity (particularly, a low death rate from heart disease) if they reside in areas with relatively high levels of calcium and/or magnesium ions in the drinking water.

Acid conditions precede the production of large concentrations of oxygen free radicals in body cells. Acid conditions increase the strength of oxygen free radical reactions (activated oxygen species reactions), which are involved in the processes of cell injury and cell death. Cell injury and cell death from oxygen free radical reactions initiate many diseases of body organs, including diseases of joints, kidney, lung, and heart. These free radical reactions are involved also in the initiation of cancer and the processes of aging and senescence. It is considered that normal adults eating ordinary Western diets have chronic, low-grade acidosis, which increases with age. This excess acid, or acidosis, is considered to contribute to many diseases and to the aging process. Acidosis occurs often when the body cannot produce enough bicarbonate ions (or other alkaline compounds) to neutralize the acids in the body formed from metabolism.

It is known also that bicarbonate ions and other alkaline compounds prevent the harmful effects of acid on bone and prevent or retard muscle catabolism. In addition, the avoidance and prevention of acid conditions in the body are highly essential for optimum health because the activities of almost all enzyme systems in the body are affected detrimentally by excess acid. Acid conditions in the body alter nearly all cell, organ, and body functions. This leads to aberrations in homeostasis, and contributes to the pathogenesis of many diseases.

Acid conditions in the body alter the net charge on protein surfaces and alter the hydrogen bonding of proteins. As acid conditions increase, acidic amino acid side chains on proteins become protonated. This results in alterations in the charges on the surface of proteins. These charge alterations have a dramatic effect on protein stability, which impacts on enzyme and structural protein function. When we consume water with sodium bicarbonate, the bicarbonate ions enter the body and help to neutralize the production of acid from carbon dioxide and other sources in body cells. The ingested bicarbonate enhances the large amount of natural bicarbonates produced in the body each day by the kidneys, brain, pancreas, red blood cells, and other tissues. Indeed, the kidneys alone produce about two hundred and fifty grams (about half a pound) of bicarbonate per day in an attempt to neutralize acid in the body. In addition, the brain produces each day about half a liter of cerebrospinal fluid, which is rich in bicarbonate. The pancreas produces each day about three liters of pancreatic fluid which is rich in bicarbonate.

The human body goes to great lengths to neutralize the production of acid from carbon dioxide in body cells. Indeed, the fastest known enzyme in the world exists in human cells to catalyze the rapid production of bicarbonate, in order to neutralize acid. This enzyme, carbonic anhydrase, is ubiquitous in the body and occurs in most cells and tissues. Each molecule of carbonic anhydrase enzyme catalyzes the production of one thousand to one million bicarbonate ions per second.

Scientific Findings

Medical scientists in the Department of Molecular Biology at the University of Occupational and Environmental Health—School of Medicine in Fukuoka, Japan have identified four major types of pH regulator: the proton pump, the sodium-proton exchanger family, the bicarbonate transporter family, and the monocarboxylate transporter family. Understanding pH regulation in tumor cells suggests that the bicarbonate often used with cancer patients for a variety of reasons would be effective inducing tumor-specific apoptosis.

> *Cancer tissues have a much higher concentration of toxic chemicals, pesticides, etc then do healthy tissues.*

In 1973, a study conducted by the Department of Occupational Health at Hebrew University—Hadassah Medical School in Jerusalem found that when cancerous breast tissue is compared with non-cancerous tissue from elsewhere in the same woman's body, the concentration of toxic chemicals such as DDT and PCBs was "much increased in the malignant tissue compared to the normal breast and adjacent adipose tissue."[4] This should say something to the oncologists of the world about chemical etiologies that are going undiagnosed and untreated.

In late stages of acidic pH, we need to turn to the most alkaline minerals to increase our throw weight of alkalinity into cancer cells. Mass spectrographic and isotope studies have shown that potassium, rubidium, and especially cesium are most efficiently taken up by cancer cells. This uptake was enhanced by Vitamins A and C, as well as salts of zinc and selenium. The quantity of cesium taken up was sufficient to raise the cell to the 8 pH range.[5]

Alkalinity and pH

Alkalinity and pH are related to each other, but are not quite the same. The idea that alkalinity is separate from pH (which is by 'coincidence' called either acid or alkaline) is a myth, though *pH and alkalinity are two different measurable parameters of water.* Even though the pH can be very high, we find that unmineralized water has little ability to neutralize acid in the stomach to initiate the production of bicarbonate in the bloodstream. Alkalinity is important because it protects or buffers against rapid pH changes.

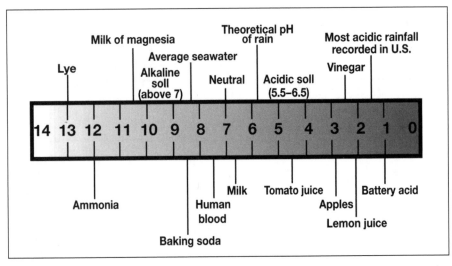

Figure 11.1. Measure of Alkalinity Levels

Alkalinity is a measure of the buffering capacity of water—its ability to resist sudden changes in pH. pH is a measure of how acidic or basic water is.

Alkalinity is the water's capacity to resist changes in pH that would make the water more acidic. This capacity is commonly known as "buffering capacity." For example, if you add the same weak acid solution to two vials of water—both with a pH of 7, but one with no buffering power (for example, zero alkalinity) and the other with buffering power (e.g. an alkalinity of 50 mg/l)—the pH of the zero alkalinity water will immediately drop, while the pH of the buffered water will change very little or not at all.

---

pH simply expresses the degree of hydrogen ion concentration. Alkaline means that the pH is greater than 7. Alkalinity is the true measure of acid-neutralizing capacity which includes the bicarbonate ($HCO_3{}^{-1}$), carbonate ($CO_3{}^{-2}$) and hydroxide (OH^{-1}) ions. It is measured in mg/l or ppm as $CaCO_3$.

Alkalinity of natural water is determined by the soil and bedrock through which it passes. The main sources for natural alkalinity are rocks, which contain carbonate, bicarbonate, and hydroxide compounds. Borates, silicates, and phosphates also may contribute to alkalinity. Limestone is rich in carbonates, so waters flowing through limestone regions or bedrock containing carbonates generally have high alkalinity—hence good buffering capacity. Conversely, areas rich in granites and some conglomerates and sandstones may have low alkalinity and therefore, poor buffering capacity.

A pH less than 6.5 may contribute to the corrosion of pipes and fixtures, and certainly if acid water can do this one can only wonder what it does to human innards.

The pH level of drinking water is a measure of how acidic or basic it is—pH is related to the hydrogen ions in water and stands for "potential of hydrogen." Alkalinity is a measure of the capacity of water to neutralize acids. *It measures the presence of carbon dioxide, bicarbonate, carbonate, and hydroxide ions that are naturally present in water.* At normal drinking water pH levels, bicarbonate, and carbonate are the main contributors to alkalinity. As we can see in the graph on page 108, the higher the CO_2, the more alkaline the water at a given pH.

In the chemistry of natural waters, there are several types of alkalinity that are encountered. Each of these is a measure of how much acid (H^+) is required to lower the pH to a specific level. The reason that aquarists measure alkalinity is that in normal seawater *most alkalinity consists of bicarbonate and carbonate.* Consequently, alkalinity is an indication of whether or not adequate bicarbonate is present in the water.

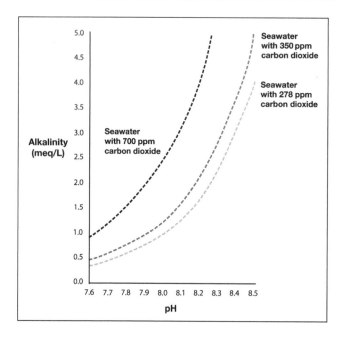

Figure 11.2.
CO_2 in Water at
a Given Alkaline
and pH

Alkaline supplied from outside the body, like drinking alkaline water,
results in a net gain of alkalinity in our body.

The main chemical species that contribute to alkalinity in seawater are bicarbonate and carbonate. The table below (from *Chemical Oceanography* by Frank Millero; 1996) shows the contribution to alkalinity from the major contributors in seawater at pH 8.

TABLE 11.1. ALKALINITY FROM THE MAJOR CONTRIBUTORS IN SEAWATER AT PH 8	
Chemical Species	Relative Contribution to Alkalinity
HCO_3^- (bicarbonate)	89.8
CO_3^- (carbonate)	6.7
$B(OH)_4^-$ (borate)	2.9
$SiO(OH)_3^-$ (silicate)	0.2
$MgOH^+$ (magnesium monohydroxylate)	0.1
OH^- (hydroxide)	0.1
HPO_4^- and PO_4^- (phosphate)	0.1

Carbon dioxide has a specific solubility in water as carbonic acid (H_2CO_3). At any given pH there is an exact mathematical relationship between H_2CO_3 and both bicarbonate and carbonate. For example, at a pH of about 9.3 in freshwater (about 8.4 in seawater), the carbonate concentration is 100 times that of the carbonic acid. Alkalinity rises sharply as pH is raised. This becomes especially true above pH 8 in salt water, where there becomes an appreciable concentration of carbonate.

The theoretical relationship between carbonate alkalinity and pH for seawater (blue) and freshwater (red) equilibrated with the atmosphere (350 ppm carbon dioxide) is shown in Figure 11.3 below. Normal to high alkalinity implies adequate bicarbonate, while low alkalinity implies that it is in short supply. It is critical to see that alkalinity does not depend strictly on pH. There is a relationship between the two, but pH measures the degree of alkalinity but not its quantity. It is like the relationship between temperature and heat. You can have a paper clip heated to 10,000 degrees but it will not heat a house nearly as well as 90-degree air blown from a home heater.

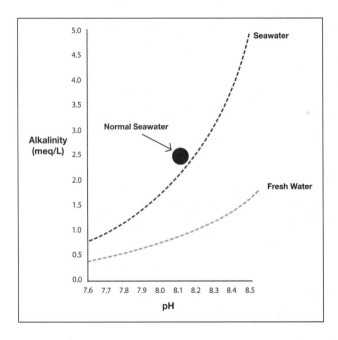

Figure 11.3
Carbonate Alkalinity and pH in Seawater and Freshwater

Alkalinity measures the concentrations of bicarbonate, carbonate, and hydroxide ions and is expressed as an equivalent concentration of calcium carbonate ($CaCO_3$).

Alkaline ionizers do not always deliver water that is sufficiently acid-neutralizing to make a difference. Alkaline ionizer promoters equate acid-neutralizing ability with high pH. From the discussion above, we can see that it is the parameter of alkalinity that neutralizes acid, not pH levels alone. In other words, you can have high pH and little alkalinity, and you can have low pH and a lot of alkalinity (for example, sparkling mineral water). If there is only a small amount of alkaline elements (from the first two columns of the Periodic Chart), an ionizer will generate a meager quantity of acid neutralizing alkalinity—but the pH will still show as a high alkaline value (for example, 8.5 to 10.5).

The presence of calcium carbonate or other compounds, such as magnesium carbonate, contribute carbonate ions to the buffering system.

People living in low mineral areas (many city supplies and wells) think they are getting a good dose of alkalinity from their ionizers, when they would be much better off with $1/_2$ teaspoon of baking soda or a shot glass of Gerolsteiner Sparkling Water. So it will be advised for many users of water ionizers to add sodium bicarbonate to their water if they are looking for stronger healing effects.

"Alkaline water" is not the same as "water with alkalinity". For this reason, water with a pH of 6.3 (for example, sparkling mineral water) can have hundreds of times more acid-neutralizing "alkalinity" than water with an alkaline pH of 9.5 from an alkaline-ionizer.

—*Robert Slovak*

The shortcoming of ionizers is simply that the input water chemistry determines its degree of benefit in terms of acid-neutralizing alkalinity (not pH!) and negative ORP (active hydrogen). The quality of one's "raw" water resource has to have a lot to do with our decision in terms of filters and ionizers chosen.

Most practitioners promote the idea that alkaline pH implies significant acid-neutralizing capacity—but that is not always correct. There are good reasons to suggest that those who have ionizer machines should add extra alkalinity (bicarbonate)—if the mineral content of their water supply is low. When the source water is low in minerals (most public drinking waters are low in minerals, especially magnesium and bicarbonate) re-mineralization becomes critical.

> *Alkaline solutions, at about pH 8.5 has been shown to overtly increase the antioxidant effect by up to 60 percent, relative to the same compound tested in a near biological pH of 7.4.[6]*

Sang Whang, one of the world's great experts on reversing aging, reminds us that, "The ingredients in the stomach cell that make hydrochloric acid (HCl) are carbon dioxide (CO_2), water (H_2O), and sodium chloride (NaCl) or potassium chloride (KCl)."

$$NaCl + H_2O + CO_2 = HCl + NaHCO_3, \text{ or}$$
$$KCl + H_2O + CO_2 = HCl + KHCO_3$$

Wang says, "In order to digest food and kill the kinds of bacteria and viruses that come with the food, the inside of our stomach is acidic. The stomach pH value is maintained at around 4. When we eat food and drink water, especially alkaline water, the pH value inside the stomach goes up. When this happens, there is a feedback mechanism in our stomach to detect this, and commands the stomach wall to secrete more hydrochloric acid into the stomach to bring the pH value back to 4. So the stomach becomes acidic again. When we drink more alkaline water, more hydrochloric acid is secreted to maintain the stomach pH value."

As we can see from the above chemical equations, the byproduct of making hydrochloric acid is sodium bicarbonate ($NaHCO_3$) or potassium bicarbonate ($KHCO_3$). In response to ingestion of sodium bicarbonate or high pH alkaline water, the production of hydrochloric acid is actually increased because the stomach responds to lower the pH back down to normal acidic conditions. So as we take more alkalinity from drinking high pH and alkaline water, it forces our stomach to produce more acid (and a balancing amount of bicarbonate). The bottom line is that a net gain of alkalinity is achieved in the body, and this is extremely helpful in a body struggling to maintain equilibrium.

12. *Sodium Bicarbonate as a World Class Anti-Fungal*

Sodium bicarbonate acts as a powerful, natural and safe antifungal agent,[1] which when combined with iodine, would probably cover the entire spectrum of microbial organisms. The efficacy of sodium bicarbonate against certain bacteria and fungi[2] has been documented.

Years ago, I worked with a man in Hawaii who has an out of control Candida infection in his intestines, something easily diagnosed as intestinal cancer. He was putting a cup of bicarbonate into a quart of water and using the mixture in his daily enemas. Bicarbonate is an excellent antifungal. "Even patients who had been committed to mental hospitals have been helped by anti-fungal therapy. Other puzzling immunologic diseases, including multiple sclerosis, rheumatoid arthritis, and lupus erythematosus, have responded better when attention was given to reduction of yeast and immune stress. A wide spectrum of allergic disorders, from classical hay fever to chronic, delayed-onset type of food allergy and petrochemical sensitivity have improved following anti-yeast therapy," says Dr. Elmer M. Cranton.[3]

Why is this important? Because some people believe that cancer is a fungus, or as clinical reality dictates, people with late-stage cancer usually have late stage infections, fungal in nature, which need to be treated with anti-fungal medications. No matter what we believe, we have every reason to suspect that when we successfully treat fungal infections in cancer patients, they will improve.

Sodium bicarbonate is a proven antifungal in agriculture, resolving fungal issues in vegetation, including many destructive diseases, such as anthracnose, powdery mildew, black spot in crops, and horticultural industries. It has also been successfully used to protect crops from fungus during storage.

Treating Cancer

Traditional anti-fungal drugs are ineffective in treating tumors because the solid colonies can be attacked only on the surface of their volume, and after the first administrations they become resistant. A solid tumor with fungal infection is powerful and they resist attack and adapt quite readily to pharmaceutical drugs. After all, fungi love to chew on rocks, and they eat mercury for breakfast, so you have to hit them correctly in an all-out frontal attack with sodium bicarbonate and iodine.

Most of us have a concept of cancer that has been programmed into us through years of constant and deliberate misinformation. All we can think of is our DNA strands losing control of themselves, creating colonies of human cells running amuck. Tell someone that their cancer is a yeast or fungi invasion and they will look at you like you are a nut. But a major US scientist said, cancer—always believed to be caused by genetic cell mutations—can in reality be caused by infections from viruses, bacteria, yeasts, molds, and fungus parasites. "I believe that, conservatively, 15 to 20 percent of all cancer is caused by infections; however, the number could be larger—maybe double," said Dr. Andrew Dannenberg, director of the Cancer Center at New York-Presbyterian Hospital/Weill Cornell Medical Center." Dr. Dannennberg made the remarks in a speech in December 2007 at the annual international conference of the American Association for Cancer Research.

We know that liver cancer is often caused by chronic hepatitis B and C. Human papillomavirus (HPV) is linked to cervical, throat, and oral cancer (oropharyngeal carcinoma).A form of gastric cancer, called adenocarcinoma, and a form of lymphoma, called MALT lymphoma, have been linked to Helicobacter pylori bacteria. Bladder cancers are often caused by chronic infection with Schistosome parasites. Today we need to know how inflammation caused by infections leads to a variety of cancers.

Sodium Bicarbonate as a Remedy

Dr. Tullio Simoncini states, "At the moment, against fungi, there is no useful remedy other than, in my opinion, sodium bicarbonate. The anti-fungins that are currently on the market, in fact, do not have the ability to penetrate the masses (except perhaps early administrations of azoli or of amfotercin B delivered parenterally), since they are conceived to act only at a stratified level of epithelial type. In order to achieve the most detrimental effect on the tumors, the sodium bicarbonate must be put in direct contact with the damaged tissue. It is also possible to put specific catheters (port-a-cath) in the arteries that run to the different conventional endoscope methods. Furthermore there can be used clysters, drip infusions, irrigations, and infiltrations at the places where the tumor has grown."

Dr. Simoncini says, "It is useful to consider the extreme sensitivity of fungi to saline and electrolytic solutions. These solutions, because of their extreme capacity for diffusion, are able to reach all the myceliar biological expressions, including the most infinitesimal ones. Salts and bicarbonates, by making the "terrain" completely inorganic, eliminate the slightest organic fonts that fungi could use for nourishment. In this context, sodium bicarbonate, which is currently used in children's oral candidoses, appears to be a simple and handy weapon capable of uprooting, inhibiting, or attenuating any neoplastic formation wherever it is possible to easily apply it."

Antifungals work by exploiting differences between mammalian and fungal cells to kill off the fungal organism without dangerous effects on the host. Unlike bacteria, both fungi and humans are eukaryotes. Thus fungal and human cells are similar at the molecular level. This means it is more difficult to find and attack a weakness in fungi that does not also exist in human cells. So if you attack the fungus, you may also attack the human cells the fungus lives on. Consequently, there are often side-effects to these drugs. Some of these side-effects can be life-threatening.

After an increase in local pH was noted, sodium bicarbonate was used to treat vaginitis to provide symptomatic relief for women. Fungal vaginitis, one of the common female vaginal diseases with a high morbidity rate, is difficult to effect a radical cure. In the US, more than 75 percent women suffer from fungal vaginitis at least once in their life, and about 5 percent of adult women suffer from repeated fungal vaginal infection. It is difficult to treat.[4] The main clinical symptoms of these vaginal diseases include vulval pruritus, vaginal pain, leukorrhagia, dyspareunia, and urodynia. Therefore, this disease is harmful to the health of women as well as their quality of life.

Dr. Robert Young states, "Bacteria, yeast/fungi, and mold are not the cause of a cancerous condition, but are the result and the evidence of cells and tissues biologically transforming from a healthy state to an unhealthy state." Dr. Young astutely observed that, "over-acidification of the body leads to the development of chronic yeast, fungal infections, and ultimately a cancerous condition of the cells and tissues. Fungal infection deep in the body is a serious health problem that can be fatal."

There is a food connection to cancer, but only to its connection with contaminating fungi and the mycotoxins which those fungi produce.
—*Dr. A.V. Costantini*

Antibiotics increase the risk of incident and fatal breast cancer or any type of cancer.[5] This finding is partially explained by the fact that most of our antibiotics are derived from fungi—they are fungal byproducts, or "myco" —toxins. Remember how we get penicillin from the Penicillium mold? Or how we get alcohol from brewer's yeast, or Saccharomyces cerevisiae?

Alcohol—linked to 50 different types of cancer (Costantini, Fungalbionics Series. 1998–99)—is a mycotoxin. That same book by Costantini tells us that two or more cumulative month's use of antibiotics in one's life increases the risk of lymphoma by 40 percent. "Certainly, physicians would not believe such a risk exists for penicillin, an antibiotic given to billions of humans. However, it is by definition a mycotoxin and mycotoxins do cause cancer." (Costantini, et al. 1998).

Both cancer cells and fungi can metabolize nutrients in the absence of oxygen (anaerobically). Both must have sugar in order to survive. Both can be impacted by antifungal medicines.[6] Both will die in the absence of sugar.[7] "Mycotoxins have proven to be very toxic and harmful, and it is no wonder that many inhabitants of mold-infested spaces are constantly ill. This illness is mainly upper respiratory tract infections, lethargy, constant headaches, nausea, and a general ill feeling. Inhabiting these living spaces for a considerable period may lead to cancer."[8]

Contributing to this explosion are the excessive amounts of toxins and pollutants, high stress lifestyles that zap the immune system, poor quality pesticide, junk food, irradiated genetically modified pathogens, electromagnetic stress, lights, and just about everything that wasn't here 200 years ago. All these weaken the immune system and alter the internal environment in the body to an environment that promotes the growth of cancer/fungal colonies.

Fungi easily grow in the body after the part of the immune system that controls the fungi (for example, kills it) has been compromised—compromised for example by heavy metals, pesticides, emotional shocks, and antibiotics. If the immune system is 100 percent intact, then fungi should not grow in the body. The part of the immune system that is most responsible for attacking fungi is the neutraphil function.

Dr. Milton White believed that cancer is a chronic, infectious, fungus disease. He was able to find fungal spores in every sample of cancer tissue he studied.[9] Pathogenic albicans (chronic candidiasis, more commonly known as candida or thrush) is generally caused by drug use—particularly antibiotic drug use, poor diet, lowered immunity, and metals like mercury from dental amalgams. Mercury will promote the growth of Candida, as it adsorbs the mercury.

> *Two studies found an association between exposure to mercury and acute leukemia. On the basis of the available human and animal data, the International Agency for Research on Cancer and the U.S. Environmental Protection Agency has classified methyl mercury as a "possible" human carcinogen.*
> *—National Academy of Science10*

According to the observations made by the internationally recognized medical researcher, Dr. Yoshiaki Omura, all cancer cells have mercury in them. Support for this idea comes from Dr. Hans Nolte who states, "The wave spectrum of mercury contains more than thirteen wavelengths, whereas only one or two frequencies or wavelengths are usually observed for the other heavy or noble metals." Dr. Omura's clinical observation concludes that one of the primary reasons cancer returns is because residual mercury reignites a pathological environment, even after surgery, chemotherapy, radiation, and alternative therapies report a positive effect.[11]

Treating Fungus and Cancer Together

According to *The Home Medical Encyclopedia*, in 1963 about one-half of all Americans suffered from an "unrecognized" systemic fungal condition. Far more Americans suffer from fungal infections today, as antibiotics, hormone replacement therapies, and birth control pills continue to be consumed like cotton candy.

> *In my practice I've noticed that clients who have chronic sub-clinical viral, bacterial or yeast/fungal infections accumulate and retain heavy metals in their bodies. It's interesting to note that these chronic infections bind to toxic metals so effectively that no chelating agent is able to remove them.*
> *—Dr. Ted Edwards*

The Peter MacCallum Cancer Centre in East Melbourne spoke of cancer patients who died from fungal infections in its intensive care unit.[12] After a cycle of antibiotic use, the candida/yeast/fungus overgrowth that comes in its wake becomes lethal. Cancer is defined as malignant tumor of disorderly cells that have the potential of nearly unlimited growth. These uncontrolled cells expand locally and/or metastasize (spread destructively) to other tissues and organs. Clearly this can define a yeast or fungus colony as well as normal cells losing control of their own reproductive growth.

Dr. H. Takeuchi et al in Japan analyzed 20 cases of urinary fungal infection. Candida albicans was the most prevalent of the fungi affecting the urinary tract. Torulopsisglabrata and Candida tropicalis were also prevalent. Antibiotics, indwelling catheter and obstructive uropathy were the most prevalent predisposing factors of the fungal infection. In 20 cases of fungal infection studied, 5 cases were cured only by elimination of the predisposing factors. Fifteen cases were treated and *resolved by administration of sodium bicarbonate*, 5-fluorocytosine, and/or irrigation with amphotericin B. But one case of bilateral renal torulopsiosis developed into renal failure, and 4 cases died of the primary disease.[13]

Children with cancer often require pediatric intensive care; and thanks to such care, many of them have been able to overcome their leukemia. Intensive care resources are used even in incurable cases, and those resources include sodium bicarbonate, which is a staple in such units. It is used to relieve immediate symptoms and improve quality of life.

Practically all organs may be affected by cancer or by its treatment. The main complications include infections, hematological problems, and electrolyte/metabolic disturbances. Intensive care therapy is necessary to correct organic dysfunctions (cardiovascular, respiratory, renal, gastrointestinal, and neurologic). Intensive care therapy in children with cancer is not always futile. There has been a reduction in mortality and an improvement in the quality of life for these children, in the medium and long terms. There is something being done to these children that is improving their survival rates.

In 1999, Meinolf Karthaus, MD watched three different children with leukemia suddenly go into remission upon receiving a triple antifungal drug cocktail for their "secondary" fungal infections.[14]

Dr. Roberto Sapolnik indicates that the interaction between the intensive care team and oncologists allows for the solution of extremely life-threatening situations for children with leukemia. He writes, "Neoplasms are the second most common cause of death in children aged between 1 and 15 years throughout most of the world, being outrivaled only by accident-related traumas. Leukemia is the most frequent type of childhood cancer, followed (in decreasing order) by brain tumor, lymphomas, sarcoma, and ectodermal tumors. Tremendous development has been made in cancer treatment in the last twenty years, especially with the advent of new chemotherapy drugs, radiotherapy, and bone marrow transplant. However, these new therapies may cause several side effects and compromise almost all the organic functions. Cancer itself may cause clinical complications with immediate life threat, such as spontaneous tumor lysis syndrome or tumor compression, causing renal insufficiency or intestinal obstruction. Children with cancer often require pediatric intensive care; and thanks to such care, many of them have been able to overcome the most acute phase of the disease."

Something is happening in the intensive care wards that are not being explained or understood. Perhaps the intensive care staffs are unwittingly killing off the yeast, fungi, and molds (cancer) that are choking off the life force of these unfortunate children. If leukemia turns out to be a fungal infection of white blood cells called leukocytes, then all will be explained.

Fungi Mycotoxins Poison Us

Although there are millions of species of fungi, only about 400 species of fungi make mycotoxins that are capable of causing human illness. Only one, a mycotoxin from the fungi Aspergillus called aflatoxin, is routinely tested in our food supply.[15] It is tested in corn, peanuts, and other products. A study published in January 2002 in *The Journal of the American Medical Association (JAMA)* states virtually all of our corn supply, and much of our peanut and grain supply, is impregnated with mycotoxins.

The various foods which are documented to cause prostate cancer, share little in common, except that they are all high on the list of fungal mycotoxin contaminated foods. The carcinogenic mycotoxin most often encountered is aflatoxin. Aflatoxin, a recognized potent carcinogenic mycotoxin, causes normal human breast cells to become cancerous. Tumor tissues have higher aflatoxin-adduct levels than do normal tissue from the same individual. The presence of carcinogenic aflatoxin within the cancer tissue implicates aflatoxin as a cause of breast cancer. Le et al. (1986), in a French case-control study of 1,010 breast cancer cases and 1,950 controls with nonmalignant diseases, found that breast cancer was found to be associated with increased frequency of mold-fermented cheese consumption.

Dr. Holland says, "Although aflatoxin is the most carcinogenic substance on the planet, ochratoxin beats it ten times over in terms of its toxicity and the damage it inflicts on the human body.[16] Despite this, the USDA does not screen for ochratoxin. Other countries screen for up to 15 of the most common mycotoxins, including zearalenone, fumonisin, and the aforementioned ochratoxin. Although these mycotoxins are common in our food supply, the USDA does not screen for their presence either.[17]

Incidentally, mold-generated zearalenone mimics estrogen, which can throw a victim's entire hormonal systems off balance. It is found in high concentrations in North America."[18]

While cooking will kill fungi, their mycotoxins remain unaffected by heat. So mycotoxins existing in grains, milk, and animals fed them (livestock) will be carried to our dinner tables. We are eating fungi in our grains, meats, fruits, processed foods, and taking them in our medicines, and even breathing them in from the air around us.

Fungus, Food and Diabetes—Antecedents to Cancer

Doug A. Kaufman and David Holland, M.D., in their book *Infectious Diabetes*, present a compelling account of how fungi may be the underlying cause of diabetes and its complications, as well as many other auto-immune disorders. The premise behind the book is that, contrary to being a genetic disease, diabetes is actually caused by microbes and toxins in the foods we eat. Fungal infections are presented as the primary cause, not a secondary infection, and that fungal infections are only partly due to antibiotic use. This book presents the other part of the story, the constant mercury exposure and dramatic nutritional deficiencies, especially that of magnesium.

Fungi are found in foods that we eat every day. Our primary concern is the long-term effects of ingesting food contaminated with low levels of mycotoxins," and that carcinogenic toxins, such as aflatoxin, a by-product of the Aspergillus molds, is a "common contaminant of peanuts, soybeans, grains, and cassava. It's a "frequent contaminant of wheat and corn." Without a properly-functioning immune system, we're at risk of succumbing to various infectious and chronic diseases. Fungi invade our grain food supply because grains—a source of carbohydrates-are their favorite food.

Fungi are parasites whose mission is to invade a larger host. Given a chance, they will alter our body chemistries to suit their needs. Both type one and type-2 diabetes, as well as gestational diabetes, may stem from specific fungi and their mycotoxins entering our systems and setting up residence by destroying the body's ability to lower blood sugar, which is the food they need and want to proliferate. Once the pancreatic beta cells are destroyed by these mycotoxins, insulin is no longer produced, (Type-1, absolute insulin deficiency) or the remaining beta cells still produce insulin, but it is ineffective in bringing down blood sugar (Type-2). In either type, sugar remains elevated in the bloodstream giving fungi the perfect opportunity to feed, proliferate, and possibly go on to infect other organs and eventually cause cancer or be the cancer that is life-threatening.

A recent Japanese study suggests that fungal mold toxins have the ability to signal the beta cells in the pancreas to shut off by killing them.

In their refutation of the theory of autoimmunity, Kaufman and Holland explain that in Type-1 diabetes it is entirely plausible that an invading fungi has altered beta cells, remained undetected, yet set off the body's immune defense system, which are unable to destroy the offending fungi, allowing them to continue to invade other beta cells and progressively lead to total destruction and a complete lack of insulin.

Dr. A.V. Constantini, former head of the WHO Collaborating Center for Mycotoxins in Food, has spent 20 years studying and collecting data on the role fungi and mycotoxins play in devastating diseases. In his research, he found a number of fungi that demonstrate specific toxicity to the pancreas.

The origin of many diseases that are referred to as having an unknown etiology or idiopathic is that it is in the "food" we eat and the many mycotoxins found in our daily diet.
—*Professor M.J. Dumanov*

The Aspergillus mold toxin, aflatoxin B1, inhibits the breakdown of both glucose, or simple sugar, and glycogen. Fungi, and the mycotoxins they produce, can also impact our genetic code, causing alterations that are found in a majority of cancers, reports Doug Kaufman. "Altering a cell's DNA amounts to changing the environmental code of that cell. Once changed the cell may respond differently—or not at all to outside *hormones and enzymes that normally stimulate it to perform necessary functions. As* one example of genetic alteration, aflatoxin B1 causes a break in DNA that alters the p53 tumor expression gene. Changes in this particular gene allow the cell to proliferate out of control. So it's no accident that this same mycotoxin can also go on to cause liver cancer."

Fungi and their mycotoxins manipulate their hosts on the cellular level, and prevent us from defending ourselves by subverting the immune system.

The Aspergillus mold toxins are commonly found in corn, wheat, peanuts, barley, and other grains. Pennicillium and Aspergillus mold produce a mycotoxn called ochratoxin, which causes apoptosis (cell death) and depletes our stores of gluthatione (GSH), which is an important toxin-neutralizing substance, also known to have a significant role in insulin sensitivity. Diabetics typically test low in glutathione levels.

Uric Acid

Uric Acid was discovered to cause diabetes in 1949, by Mervyn Griffiths. Alloxan, now used to make laboratory rats diabetic for research purposes is formed from uric acid. Urea and uric acid are always found together in the urine, along with a small amount of alloxan. Alloxan appears to be the intermediate stage in the conversion of uric acid into urea by oxidation. Uric acid or alloxan alone in small amounts did not cause a diabetic condition if the glutathione levels remained at normal levels in the lab animals tested. Sacchromyces yeast produces uric acid.(Svlhia,1963), and in 1976 after two children dying from diabetes were found to be infected with Cryptococcus fungi, further studies were done by injecting Cryptococcus directly into the pancreatic arteries. Necrosis (cell death) in the Islets of Langerhans resulted.

Cryptococcus fungi also produce alloxan, a uric acid byproduct. Further studies through the years confirmed alloxan's damage to the pancreatic islet cells. (Pogo,1980) and in 1990 Coleman et al fed mice a diet of 10 percent brewers yeast, and diabetes resulted. In the 1980s, it was found that other alloxan-like metabolites of uric acid were diabetogenic, some even more so than alloxan.

Kaufman and Holland state that many fungal varieties produce uric acid which in turn produce alloxan. Alloxan is made up of allantoin and oxalic acid, and even in small quantities induces diabetes in laboratory animals. In one study they cite, it was found that rats injected with alloxan suffered a drop in the number of beta cells in their pancreases, and a corresponding sharp drop in insulin production. The rat's cholesterol and triglyceride levels shot up, as well.

Uric acid causes diabetes, heart disease, probably strokes, and renal disease, as well as gout and kidney stones. Uric acid has often been regarded as simply a "marker" of renal disease, but recently a study was conducted to clarify the role of uric acid in the kidney and determine whether uric acid might actually be a cause of renal disease.

The list of recommended foods to avoid, and are likely to contain fungi or mycotoxins includes:

- Alcoholic beverages
- Corn
- Wheat
- Barley
- Sorghum
- Peanuts

- Sugar (sugar cane and sugar beets)
- Rye
- Hard Cheeses
- Cottonseed

Going et al. (1990) found that calcium oxalate crystals are present in calcifications found in the breast tissue of patients with breast cancer. Oxalic acid (calcium oxalate crystals) in the sputum or lung specimens of patients is also an indication of an Aspergillus infection of the lung. Oxalic acid is a powerful corrosive agent, and oxalate salts are widely used for their cleaning and bleaching properties. Oxalic acid also happens to be a mycotoxin which can be produced by a number of different fungal species. Some fungi produce such large amounts of oxalic acid that they are used for commercial production of the chemical. These calcium oxalate crystals are the same as the calcium oxalate found in breast cancers. The presence of oxalates in the breast is indicative of the presence of fungi interwoven within the stages of breast cancer development. Since humans do not make oxalic acid themselves, this is an appropriate conclusion.

Death by Fungi—Scientific Findings

In *Nature* there is an essay about natural catastrophes that might overtake us. One of these focuses on the threat posed by fungus populations. "Although viruses and bacteria grab more attention, fungi are the planet's biggest killers. Of all the pathogens being tracked, fungi have caused more than 70 percent of the recorded global and regional extinctions, and now threaten amphibians, bats, and bees. The Irish potato famine in the 1840s showed just how devastating such pathogens can be. Phytophthorainfestans (an organism similar to and often grouped with fungi) wiped out as much as three-quarters of the potato crop in Ireland and led to the death of one million people." Researchers estimate that there are 1.5 to 5 million species of fungi in the world, but only 100,000 have been identified. Reports of new types of fungal infection in plants and animals have risen nearly tenfold since 1995.

Fungi are dreadful enemies. During their life cycle, fungi depend on other living beings, which must be exploited to different degrees for their feeding. Fungi can develop from the hyphae, the more or less beak-shaped specialized structures that allow the penetration of the host. The shape of a fungus is never defined; it is imposed by the environment in which the fungus develops. Fungi are capable of implementing an infinite number of modifications to their own metabolism, in order to overcome the defense mechanism of the host. These modifications are implemented through plasmatic and biochemical actions, as well as by a volumetric increase (hypertrophy) and numerical hyperplasia[19] of the cells that have been attacked.

"Fungal infections can not only be extremely contagious, but they also go hand in hand with leukemia[20]—every oncologist knows this. And these infections are devastating: Once a child who has become a bone marrow transplant recipient gets a "secondary" fungal infection, his chances of living, despite all the antifungals in the world, are only 20 percent, at best," writes Dr. David Holland.

Doug A. Kaufman wrote:

> The day I wrote this, a young lady phoned into my syndicated radio talk show. Her three-year-old daughter was diagnosed last year with leukemia. She believes antifungal drugs and natural immune system therapy has been responsible for saving her daughter's life. She is now telling others with cancer about her daughter's case. After hearing her story, a friend of hers with bone cancer asked her doctor for a prescriptive antifungal drug. To her delight, this medication, meant to eradicate fungus, was also eradicating her cancer. She dared not share this with her physician, telling him only that the antifungal medication was for a "yeast" infection. *When she could no longer get the antifungal medication, the cancer immediately grew back.* Her physician contended that a few antifungal pills surely should have cured her yeast infection. It is my contention, however, that the reason this medication worked was because she did have a yeast infection not a vaginal infection for which this medication was prescribed; a fungal infection of the bone that may have been mimicking bone cancer.

A medical textbook used to educate Johns Hopkins medical students in 1957,
Clinical and Immunologic Aspects of Fungous Diseases, declared that many
fungal conditions look exactly like cancer!
—*Doug A. Kaufmann*

The Germ That Causes Cancer

The University of Michigan Cancer Center has proclaimed that current chemotherapy targets the "wrong" cells. The Ann Arbor researchers discovered that not all cells in a tumor are equally malignant. Only a tiny minority of tumor cells are actually capable of inducing new cancers, the rest are relatively harmless. "These tumor-inducing cells have many of the properties of stem cells," said Michael F. Clarke, MD, a professor of internal medicine who directed the study. "They make copies of themselves—a process called self-renewal—and produce all the other kinds of cells in the original tumor."[21]

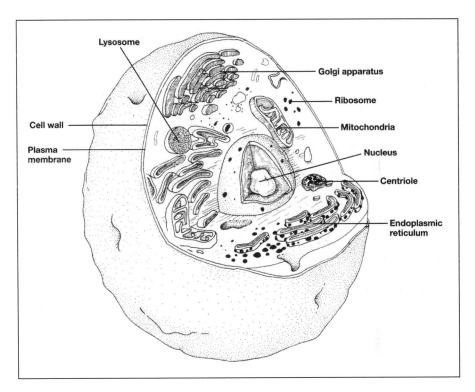

Figure 12.1 The Human Cell

According to the Mayo Clinic, cancer refers to any one of a large number of diseases characterized by the development of abnormal cells that divide uncontrollably and have the ability to infiltrate and destroy normal body tissue. This is a fact that does not depend on the various theories. The theorizing begins when we run down the usual path, thinking that cancer begins with damage (mutations) in our DNA.

Our DNA is like a set of instructions for our cells, telling them how to grow and divide. Normal cells often develop mutations in their DNA, but they have the ability to repair most of these mutations. Or, if they can't make the repairs, the cells frequently die. However, certain mutations aren't repaired, causing the cells to grow and become cancerous . . . or so the story goes. Looking at the above definition we would be perfectly correct to say that yeasts and fungi are, in human terms, abnormal cells that divide uncontrollably and have the ability to infiltrate and destroy normal body tissue.

Cancer is a biologically-induced spore (fungus) transformation disease.
Dr. Milton W. White

A new study, published in December 2012 in *Science,* could explain why almost none of the new generation of "personalized" cancer drugs is a true cure and suggests that drugs based on genetics alone will never achieve that Holy Grail of medical science. Scientists found that despite having identical genetic mutations, colorectal cancer cells behaved as differently as if they were genetic strangers. The findings challenge the prevailing view that genes determine how individual cells in a solid tumor behave, including how they respond to chemotherapy and how actively they propagate. The study suggests *DNA is not the sole driver of tumors' behavior.* "What our data are saying is, there are other biological properties that matter. Gene sequencing of tumors is definitely not the whole story when it comes to identifying which therapies will work. Our findings raise questions about the resources put into sequence, sequence, sequence," said John Dick, molecular geneticist of the Princess Margaret Cancer Centre in Toronto, who led the study. "That has led to one kind of therapeutic—molecularly-targeted drugs—but not the cures the public is being promised."

The idea that a proposed cancer germ could have more than one form is a threat
to doctors and some microbiologists. Indeed the cancer germ has been described
as having a virus-like and fungus-like, as well as a mycoplasma-like phase.
—Dr. Alan Cantwell, The Cancer Microbe

"In some cases, the aggressive power of fungi is so great as to allow it, with only a cellular ring made up of three units, to tighten in its grip, capture and kill its prey in a short time notwithstanding the prey's desperate struggling. Fungus, which is the most powerful and the most organized micro-organism known, seems to be an extremely logical candidate as a cause of neoplastic proliferation," Dr. Simoncini says, "Candida albicans clearly emerges as the sole candidate for tumoral proliferation."

Fungi are heterotrophs, meaning that they secrete digestive enzymes and absorb the resulting soluble nutrients from whatever they are growing on.

Fungi Love Mercury

Research being driven by Dundee life scientists is revealing remarkable abilities of fungi to interact with minerals and metals. Led by Professor Geoffrey Gadd in the College of Life Sciences, the research explores *the unique taste that fungi seems to have for rock and heavy metal.*[22] This environmental science has demonstrated the power of fungi to eat through concrete and to absorb heavy metals such as mercury and uranium in the environment. Fungi will live almost anywhere. They have been found growing in the harshest of environments, in the desert and in Polar Regions, in the sea and on rocks. "The fact that fungi interact with heavy metals has potentially important consequences for human activity. Fungi also play a significant, if often overlooked, role in the degradation of rocks and stone—including building materials," Professor Gadd said. "Despite this, their role as agents of environmental change has not been fully appreciated."

Evidence in studying wildlife has shown a strong relationship between fungi and mercury accumulation.[23] Medical scientists at Arizona State University tell us that *antibiotic use is known to almost completely inhibit excretion of mercury* in rats due to alteration of gut flora.[24] Thus, higher use of oral antibiotics—in children destined to contract autism—may have reduced their ability to excrete mercury. Antibiotics, such as tetracycline, can greatly increase yeast in the colon after only a few days. The extensive use of antibiotics will make the condition of Candida much worse because it reduces heavy metal excretion, which is a food source for the yeast like organism and also killing the beneficial bacteria at the same time.

Dr. Elmer Cranton says that, "Yeast overgrowth is partly iatrogenic (caused by the medical profession) and can be caused by antibiotics and cortisone medications. A diet high in sugar also promotes overgrowth of yeast. A highly refined diet common in industrialized nations not only promotes growth of yeast, but is also deficient in many of the essential vitamins and minerals needed by the immune system. Chemical colorings, flavorings, preservatives, stabilizers, and emulsifiers add more to stress on the immune system."

13. *Nebulizing Bicarbonate and Other Medicinals*

Sometimes very sick people or even animals with a lung ailment do better when taking drugs by nebulization as opposed to orally, because then the embattled system doesn't need to go through breaking down the medications in the stomach and then delivering them to the lungs through the bloodstream. With nebulization medicines get sprayed directly onto the lung tissues where they can most easily be absorbed locally by the lung and brachial cells. Dr. Shallenberger says, "A nebulizer is able to convert a liquid into tiny bubbles that are so tiny that they can only be seen under a microscope. When these bubbles come out of the nebulizer, they are so small that they look just like smoke. And that's the magic of a nebulizer. The bubbles are so small that they can be inhaled deep down into the deepest regions of the lungs without any discomfort or irritation. It's a great way for asthmatics to get the medication they need to open up their lungs."

Few practitioners consider the systemic effects of nebulizers. When we hear from patients using nebulizers with pharmaceuticals that it makes them feel the side effects just as badly as when the doctors were giving the same drug intravenously in the hospital, we are actually hearing that the medicines are not only being delivered to the lungs, but also being delivered directly into the blood stream and systemically into the rest of the body. This is very important to understand and appreciate because it opens a wonderful delivery system that is important for certain populations like infants, children, intensive care patients, and to all those who are trying to care for themselves or loved ones at home. And that's when Dr. Shallenberger thought, "Why not use the nebulizer delivery system to deliver treatments not just to the lungs, but to the whole body?"

Using the Nebulizer Delivery System

The great strength of nebulizers though is their capability of delivering medications and moisture directly to the tracheobronchial tree. Contrary to other treatment options, higher concentrations in respiratory secretions can be achieved with aerosol therapy. With the use of this localized delivery system, effective antimicrobials can have a direct effect on surface organisms in the bronchial system.

- Nebulization thins secretions and mucus making it easier to expel pulmonary secretions.

- Nebulization makes coughing easier while lessening the need to cough.

- Nebulization keeps your windpipe & trachea lining and stoma moist and healthy.

- Nebulization moistens the air that goes into your lungs.

- Nebulization hydrates & moisturizes your nasal passages, mouth and throat.

Nebulizers are good for young children, people who have trouble using metered dose inhalers, and people who have severe asthma. Within 10 to 15 minutes, the medication is used up and symptoms are gone or prevented for six to eight hours. Even babies can breathe the mist, and nebulizer treatments are fast becoming pediatrician-approved alternatives to over-prescribed antibiotics.

Several devices are available to create the drug aerosol particles. These include jet nebulizers, ultrasonic nebulizers, metered-dose inhalers, and dry powder inhalers through which particles can reach the upper and lower respiratory tracts and be quickly absorbed into the bloodstream. Aerosolized drugs have several advantages, including quick onset of action and low incidence of systemic adverse effects.[1] Delivery of aerosolized medications typically does not cause pain to the patient, and it is frequently a more convenient method of drug delivery. Studies show that the device used really doesn't matter, as long as it's used properly. All methods work just as well when the correct technique is used.[2] Nebulizing is generally carried out for ten, twenty, or thirty minutes each time, and for best results one may need to nebulize up to five times a day.

Transdermal medicine delivers medications to the exact site of injury, pain or disease. Transdermal medicine applied through a nebulizer is ideal for direct treatment to the lungs. Transdermal methods of delivery are increasingly being used because they allow the absorption of medicine directly through the skin, and in this case we conceptualize the lungs as an inner skin. Such treatments ensure that medications reach the site of needed action directly; bypassing the stomach and liver, meaning a much greater percentage of the active ingredient gets to target tissues.

At the Ohio State University Medical Center, pharmacists, respiratory therapists, and pulmonologists endorse what they call off-label nebulization. Off-label nebulization is a rapidly growing area of patient care, and in time, new research and practical experience will bring us much more information on how magnesium and other agents like sodium bicarbonate, iodine, peroxide, and glutathione can be administered directly into the lungs for many difficult-to-treat conditions. Even DMSO has been used in veterinarian medicine, and naturopaths have used Tea Tree Oil from Australia, which is used topically as fungicide antiseptic and germicide. Eucalyptus oil has also been used forever because it is a known bronchial-dilator.

Nebulized Bicarbonate

The bronchial secretions during attack of bronchial asthma are acidic. The acidity imparts stickiness to the secretions and moreover there is high level of neuraminic acid, which possibly correlates with the stickiness. Thus sodium bicarbonate is an excellent choice for nebulization, offering its powerful and instant pH changing effects. Dr.Tullio Simoncini recommends aerosol use of bicarbonate for lung and bronchial adenocarcinoma. He recommends putting one tablespoon sodium bicarbonate in $1/_2$ liter water and inhaling it with a fast inhaler in half an hour. Six days on six days off when in IV break phases.

Dr. Lewis Nelson, a specialist in emergency medicine says, "Nebulized sodium bicarbonate has been shown to provide symptomatic relief in patients exposed to chlorine, and it is probably useful with all irritant gases that liberate acid. Through a neutralization reaction, the damaging effects of the acids are limited. Nebulized sodium bicarbonate should be used in concentrations of less than 2 percent (which generally means about a 4:1 dilution of standard 8 percent sodium bicarbonate)."[3]

General Instructions

The basic aim of a nebulizer is to facilitate a faster and more effective absorption of the medicine. This is achieved by breaking down the liquid medicine into very fine particles, which is inhaled by the patient.

1. The first step is to add the liquid medicine to the cup attached to the device. It is important to understand that these devices accept medicine in the liquid form only, and medicine should be added at the time of usage and not before that. If the doctor has prescribed more than one medicine for nebulization, make sure if they can be mixed together or whether they should be taken separately.

2. Once the medicine is put in the cup, close the cup and connect its tube to the air compressor.

3. Turn the compressor on, and when the compressed air reaches the nebulizer cup, it will vaporize the medicine, creating a mist.

4. The mist is inhaled by the patient, through the mouthpiece or face mask. Take deep breaths and inhale the vapor completely.

5. Tap the cup regularly to ensure the right dispensation of medicine, and don't remove the mask until the medicine is used up completely. It will take about 10 to 20 minutes to finish nebulization, depending on what type of medicinal is used.

6. Turn on the air pump, and a mist will come from the mouthpiece. Place the mouthpiece in your mouth and breathe in slowly.

7. At full inhalation, hold your breath for a 2 to 4 count to allow absorption in the lungs. If you are treating colds or sinus problems, you can also alternate breathing through your nose.

Most of the published research about nebulization is on standard usages like asthma, but this delivery system can be used to treat lung cancer, pneumonia, tuberculosis, as well as the influenza, chemical poisoning, and actually any syndrome requiring the administration of a medicinal. For pediatricians and parents, nebulizers are a God send because our babies cannot pop pills, and we don't really want to be sticking needles in them every day. Transdermal medicine offers the most to the world of pediatrics, with the administration of medicines through their baths and their breathing.

14. *Oral, Transdermal, and Intravenous Use of Bicarbonate*

This chapter deals with three different delivery systems for sodium bicarbonate therapy: oral, transdermal, and intravenous. Discussed are the advantages as well as guidelines for proper dosages and preferences.

Oral Use

The great advantage to using bicarbonate orally is that one can dose during all the waking hours and receive a full course of treatment in about ten days. Anyone can drive up their pH and saturate all their cells to a much higher extent through oral and transdermal methods of administration.

Cancer patients should know that Dr. Simoncini's methods use the blood for delivery. Few doctors around the world have been able to replicate Simoncini's work, and one reason is that pH changes in the blood are limited by strictly enforced blood parameters. Exactly how high the pH is driven up in the body can be controlled simply by using pH test strips, which determines how much sodium bicarbonate to take. One can do this continuously for up to ten days, keeping the optimal anti-cancer pH level of the urine at as close to eight as possible.

Intravenous Use

Sodium Bicarbonate Injection: USP (solution of sodium bicarbonate) is administered by the intravenous route. In cardiac arrest, a rapid intravenous dose of one to two 50 mL vials (44.6 to 100 mEq) may be given initially and continued at a rate of 50 mL (44.6 to 50 mEq) every 5 to 10 minutes if necessary (as indicated by arterial pH and blood gas monitoring), to reverse the acidosis. Caution should be observed in emergencies where very rapid infusion of large quantities of bicarbonate is indicated. Bicarbonate solutions are hypertonic and may produce an undesirable rise in plasma sodium concentration in the process of correcting the metabolic acidosis. In cardiac arrest, however, the risks from acidosis exceed those of hypernatremia.

Two minutes after intubation, premature ventricular contractions, ventricular fibrillation, bradycardia, and finally cardiac arrest were recognized. An increase of serum potassium from 3.19 to 8.64 mmol/L was observed in arterial blood. The patient was immediately resuscitated with chest compressions, intravenous adrenaline, atropine, lidocaine, and sodium bicarbonate.[1]

Vigorous bicarbonate therapy is required in any form of metabolic acidosis where a rapid increase in plasma total CO_2 content is crucial, for example cardiac arrest, circulatory insufficiency due to shock or severe dehydration, and in severe primary lactic acidosis or severe diabetic acidosis. Caution should be observed in emergencies where very rapid infusion of large quantities of bicarbonate is indicated. Bicarbonate solutions are hypertonic and may produce an undesirable rise in plasma sodium concentration in the process of correcting the metabolic acidosis. In cardiac arrest, however, the risks from acidosis exceed those of hypernatremia. If you take too much bicarbonate orally, one will feel one's body resisting further ingestion.

Transdermal Use

Sodium bicarbonate injection is indicated in the treatment of metabolic acidosis which may occur in severe renal disease, uncontrolled diabetes, and circulatory insufficiency due to shock or severe dehydration, extracorporeal circulation of blood, cardiac arrest, and severe primary lactic acidosis. Sodium bicarbonate is further indicated in the treatment of drug intoxications, including barbiturates. Sodium carbonate has been found effective in treating poisoning or overdose from many chemicals and pharmaceutical drugs by negating the cardiotoxic and neurotoxic effects.[2]

Preference for Oral and Transdermal

When we employ transdermal and oral routes of administration, we are dealing with the broader issues of tissues and interstitial fluids, shifting their pH levels radically into the alkaline leaving the blood in its normally tightly controlled pH, mostly unchanged. With these methods, we do not have to worry so much about blood pH, which we never in fact want to shift too much. But despite the complications, which may be associated with intravenous sodium bicarbonate infusion, the use of this agent is a frequent necessity in patients with metabolic acidosis.

The conclusion of two physicians, who wrote reports on request of The Netherlands Health Inspectorate (Inspectievoor de Gezondheidszorg, IGZ) is that "the infusion of sodium bicarbonate to vulnerable patients is hazardous and ineffective." Oral and transdermal forms of administration are superior methods in the treatment of cancers because higher pH and oxygen levels can be maintained through continuous low cost treatment.

Guiding Dosages

The best guidance for dosages for sodium bicarbonate is provided by one's own urinary and salivary pH, which one takes in the morning or several times during the day when doing a heavy course for cancer or other serious diseases. One needs to buy inexpensive pH paper strips for this.

There is no question that plasma bicarbonate concentrations are shown to increase after oral ingestion. The most important effect of bicarbonate ingestion is the change in acid-base balance, as well as blood pH and bicarbonate concentration in biological fluids.[3] The ingestion of sodium bicarbonate as a buffering agent has been studied in various experimental designs (repeated short bout exercises or long lasting efforts) and with large dose ranges (100 to 500 mg per kg body weight, ingested or injected). In Europe, spa-goers drink bicarbonate-rich water to heal ulcers, colitis, and other gastric disorders. Ingesting bicarbonate by way of bathing stimulates circulation, possibly benefiting those with high blood pressure and moderate atherosclerosis.

While the body does have a homeostatic mechanism which maintains a constant pH 7.4 in the blood, this mechanism works by depositing and withdrawing acid and alkaline minerals from other locations, including the bones, soft tissues, body fluids and saliva. Therefore, the pH of these other tissues can fluctuate greatly.

Some believe the pH of urine remains at the acidic end of the scale because it is a reflection of the body eliminating unwanted acids and therefore, is not an accurate measure of the body's pH. The pH of saliva offers us a window through which we can see the overall pH balance in our bodies. Urinary pH quickly reflects bicarbonate administration. Saliva pH changes at a much slower rate.

Oral Dosage

Sodium bicarbonate can be used orally in doses of $1/2$ teaspoon in 4 ounces of water every two hours for pain relief, as well as gastrointestinal upset, not to exceed 7 doses per day. That's basically the receipt on every box of Arm & Hammer sold in every supermarket in the country.

Directions: for oral use from the Arm & Hammer baking soda package.

- Add $1/2$ teaspoon to $1/2$ glass (4 fluid ounces) of water every 2 hours, or as directed by physician.

- Dissolve completely in water.

- Do not take more than the following amounts in 24 hours:

  —Seven $1/2$ teaspoons.

  —Three $1/2$ teaspoons if you are over 60 years.

- Do not use the maximum dosage for more than 2 weeks.

Other Information: Each $1/2$ teaspoon contains 616 mg sodium.

There are many clinical applications for bicarbonate. "After suffering from a 4 hour long blinding headache for which nothing I took brought any relief, I tried the sodium bicarbonate, 1 teaspoon mixed in a glass of water. Within a few short minutes I could feel the headache abating, and within the hour it was completely relieved! I tried this again when another headache occurred, and it worked just as miraculously." "This is the best pain reliever of all the ones I have been trying. I am amazed that something so simple would be so potent! I haven't exceeded 7 doses a day, but wish I could. It takes the pain away for about 2 hours. Nothing seems to work more than 2 hours at a time."

One of the great questions for cancer patients, when considering oral intake of bicarbonate, is whether or not to take it with maple syrup, molasses, honey, just water, or even with lime or lemon. This question is important for patients with cancer for often their cells are starving for glucose, and perhaps the sugar acts as a kind of Trojan horse getting the cancer cells to open their mouths wide. Then the increased O_2 enters more easily.

Though I published years ago about the folk formula using maple syrup, I do not recommend that. I recommend either black strap molasses (because you don't have to cook it and because of its rich mineral status) or just with mineral water and sometimes with lemon. Bicarbonate with molasses fulfills the role of the glucose, which Dr. Simoncini always used when giving bicarbonate intravenously. Sodium bicarbonate is not a substitute for an alkaline diet, nor is it a substitute for exercise and proper breathing, which both increase a person's CO_2 levels and thus O_2 levels.

The Lemon Bicarbonate Formula

This simple formula will normalize many biological parameters, pH, ORP, phosphates, bicarbonates, and antioxidants of vitamin C. Potential miracle water.

Directions:

- One whole lemon freshly squeezed.

- Keep adding baking soda slowly, bit by bit until the fizz stops.

- Then you will add water to one half glass.

- This is often taken twice a day. To be taken once in the morning and once before bedtime, on an empty stomach.

Lemons are one of the gentlest ways to restore pH balance and alkalinity. Although lemon juice is itself acidic, the ash of lemon juice is alkaline. When you consume lemon, it neutralizes acid and makes the body more alkaline. Lemons are known to promote cleansing and rid the body of chemical and dietary toxins, boosting the immune system and supporting good health. They are central to the Master Cleanse, which is often called the Lemon Cleanse. Lemons are hardly a magic bullet, but they are a subtle, gradual way to improve pH balance.

Recommendation: Take the juice of half a lemon in a glass of warm or chilled water first thing in the morning (at least ten minutes before any food) to restore pH balance and improve digestion. Replace the white, wine, or other vinegar in home-made salad dressings with fresh-squeezed lemon juice. Most vinegars are acid ash foods, with the exception of apple cider vinegar.

Basically, lemon/lime juice idea is also good for people who fear some sodium retention issues. Since the lemon is already high on potassium, adding the sodium to neutralize the acid along the way will also create a sodium potassium balance. Use one whole freshly squeezed lemon (or lime) and keep adding the bicarbonate until the fizz stops.

Apple Cider Vinegar

Apple cider vinegar, plus baking soda, restores pH to exactly 7.0 after 2 to 3 minutes. It goes higher as you wait and settles down at about 7.3 to 7.5.

Directions:

Mix 2 tablespoons of Apple Cider Vinegar with $1/4$ teaspoons of baking soda.

Bicarbonate Enemas

"I was re-reading some of your information and it got me thinking that maybe it is time to experiment with more of your protocol. I am not feeling good at all, I have a staph-like infection with boils popping out in numerous places; any cuts and wounds are not healing and pus filled. There is lots of pain associated with these spots. Also on the left side of my large intestine I feel a blockage a few inches to the left of my belly button. This is my longest term chronic symptom for years, and it seems exacerbated right now. I can barely have a bowl movement. Even an enema just cleans out the lower few inches of the bowel and can't seem to get water past the constriction."

I started using baking soda in my enemas, and it was miraculous—the amounts and ease with which I released was profound. I use several tablespoons up to a cup of bicarbonate per quart to get the best results for me. When I added the baking soda, with warm water, things really started moving—what a relief that was."

An intravenous infusion of a solution of sodium bicarbonate reduces respiratory distress and excessive acidity of body fluids in children with life-threatening asthma flare-ups. Dr. Corinne M. P. Buysse and her colleagues point out in the medical journal *Chest* that high blood acidity, or acidosis, causes the heart to contract less strongly, reduces the effectiveness of beta-agonist bronchodilators used to treat asthma, and may stimulate rapid, shallow breathing. They explain that treatment with sodium bicarbonate has been shown to relieve bronchial spasm and restore the response to bronchodilators.

However, doctors have avoided the use of intravenous sodium bicarbonate for fear of increasing levels of carbon dioxide in the blood. Instead of injecting sodium bicarbonate, it is much simpler, safer, and vastly less expensive to simply place our patients in baths full of bicarbonate or by having them drink it, or both. Injections will always be used in emergency situations, but when bicarbonate and magnesium chloride are used correctly, we can avoid many emergency situations from developing.

15. *Bicarbonate Maple Syrup Cancer Treatment*

Forms of bicarbonate treatments are theoretically similar in principle to Insulin Potentiation Therapy (IPT). IPT treatment consists of giving doses of insulin to a fasting patient, sufficient to lower blood sugar into the 50 mg/dl. In a normal person, when you take in sugar, the insulin levels go up to meet the need of getting that sugar into the cells. In IPT, they are artificially injecting insulin to deplete the blood of all sugar, then injecting the lower doses of toxic chemo drugs when the blood sugar is driven down to the lowest possible value. During the low peak, it is said that the receptors are more sensitive and take on medications more rapidly, and in higher amounts.

The principle of taking bicarbonate with maple syrup or blackstrap molasses works in reverse to IPT in theory. The sugar is not going to end up encouraging the further growth of the cancer colonies because the increased

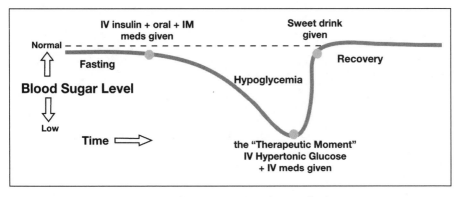

Figure 15.1 Insulin Potentiation Therapy (IPT) Curve

139

alkalinity that the baking soda yields is going to kill the cells before they have a chance to accelerate growth. Instead of artificially manipulating insulin and thus forcefully driving down blood sugar levels to then inject toxic chemo agents, we combine the sugar with the bicarbonate and present it to the cancer cells, which at first are going to love the present. But not for long! There is no science behind this, so one is on their own, but one can tell reasonably quickly if the combination suits one's body by its reactions to what is being taken.

The earliest mention of the efficacy of sodium bicarbonate being useful for cancer was in an old newspaper clipping: "There is not a tumor on God's green earth that cannot be licked with a little baking soda and maple syrup." That is the astonishing claim of controversial folk healer Jim Kelmun, who says that this simple home remedy can stop and reverse the deadly growth of cancers. His loyal patients swear by the man they fondly call Dr. Jim, and say he was a miracle worker. "Dr. Jim cured me of lung cancer," said farmer Ian Roadhouse. "Those other doctors told me that I was a goner and had less than six months to live. But the doc put me on his mixture and in a couple of months the cancer was gone. It did not even show up on the x-rays."

Dr. Jim discovered this treatment accidentally somewhere in the middle of the last century when he was treating a family plagued by breast cancer. There were five sisters in the family, and four of them had died of breast cancer. He asked the remaining sister if there was anything different in her diet, and she told him that she was partial to sipping maple syrup and baking soda. Since then, reported by a newspaper in Ashville, North Carolina, Dr. Jim dispensed this remedy to over 200 people diagnosed with terminal cancer, and amazingly, he claims of that nearly half enjoyed a complete remission of their disease.

When mixed and heated 'gently' together, the maple syrup and baking soda mix, but don't tightly bind together. The maple syrup targets cancer cells (which consume 15 times more glucose than normal cells), and the baking soda, which is dragged into the cancer cell by the maple syrup, being very alkaline forces a rapid shift in pH killing the cell. The actual formula is to mix one part baking soda with three parts (pure, 100 percent) maple syrup in a small saucepan. Stir briskly and heat the mixture for 5 minutes. With the Black Strap Molasses and honey, heating is not necessary.

Theory or Reality

This is a nice theory, but does it carry through in reality? Bicarbonate is actively transported, and perhaps as the cells open up to the sugar cell wall permeability might change. And it is not the bicarbonate itself that acts as a poison to these dangerous cells, but the shift in pH and changes in oxygen and CO_2 levels that are creating the changes. Whatever the theory it is hard to deny the testimonials that this simple combination works like magic for some people.

IPT makes cell membranes more permeable, and increases uptake of drugs into cells. The essence of IPT is that it allows cancer drugs to be given in a smaller dose, far less toxic to normal cells, while building up lethally toxic concentrations in cancer cells. Both IPT and bicarbonate maple syrup treatments theoretically try use the rabid growth mechanisms of the cancer cell against them. My suggestion if for people to try the different combinations and feel what goes down best.

Black Strap Molasses

Blackstrap molasses is a sweetener that is good for you. It is not like refined white sugar and corn syrup, which are stripped of virtually all nutrients except simple carbohydrates. Nor is it like artificial sweeteners like saccharine or aspartame, which not only provide no useful nutrients, but have been shown to cause health problems in sensitive individuals. Blackstrap molasses is a healthful sweetener that contains significant amounts of a variety of minerals that promote your health.

Blackstrap molasses is a very good source of calcium. Calcium, one of the most important minerals in the body, is involved in a variety of physiological activities essential to life. The activities include the ability of the heart and other muscles to contract, blood clotting, the conduction of nerve impulses to and from the brain, regulation of enzyme activity, and cell membrane function. Molasses is also an excellent source of copper and manganese and a very good source of potassium and even magnesium.

In addition to providing quickly assimilated carbohydrates, blackstrap molasses can increase your energy by helping to replenish iron stores. Even pregnant moms will find this a lifesaver because it can give them the iron they need, without the constipation that comes from taking iron supplements. One can put it in their oatmeal in the morning or sweeten their juices. In comparison to red meat, a well-known source of iron, blackstrap molasses provides more iron for fewer calories and is totally fat-free. Iron is an integral component of hemoglobin, which transports oxygen from the lungs to all body cells, and is also part of key enzyme systems for energy production and metabolism. Growing children and adolescents also have increased needs for iron. Just 2 teaspoons of blackstrap molasses will sweetly provide you with 13.3 percent of the daily recommended value for iron.

On the Earth Clinic site we read, "Thanks to the wonderful feedback we have received over the past eight years, blackstrap molasses appears to be making headlines as one of the best home remedies around! We have emails from our readers about blackstrap molasses curing cancerous tumors, fibroid tumors, anxiety, constipation, edema, heart palpitations, anemia, arthritic pain, joint pain, and acne, just to name a few."[1]

Chinese medicine tells us that blackstrap molasses tonifies deficiency, strengthens the spleen, lubricates lungs, stops coughs, and effectively treats stomach and abdominal pain, as well as general chi deficiency. Most westerners cannot make much sense of Chinese diagnostics, but what is being said here is that blackstrap molasses strengthens people. And when we look at its nutritional profile, we can see why.

Case in Point

Because Natural Allopathic Medicine is designed for self-administration, I include as much information in my books as possible so people can find their way without having to depend on physicians, but again it is always helpful to have good support when treating serious conditions. In this chapter I introduce Vernon Johnston, who I am happy to report is still alive and well.

Vernon reached out to me when I first began writing about sodium bicarbonate in 2007. He was diagnosed with prostate cancer with metastasis to the bones. He was going to do a cesium chloride treatment, but because his order got lost in the mail, ended up doing sodium bicarbonate (baking soda) orally, managed to get his urinary pH up to 8.5 for five days and then within two weeks was back at his oncologists office for a test, which showed his bones being cleared of his cancer.

Vernon was able to do six years ago what orthodox doctors are just thinking of getting to in the future, too late for you if you are already diagnosed with cancer. "Cancer tried to kill me, wrote Johnston. "After a struggle I said, No! Or at least I was hoping for a *no*. I turned to Cesium, but ended up with baking soda. My goal was to change my pH quickly. I knew little or next to nothing what pH, Alkaline or Acidic meant. Happily I found out."

Original Oral Treatment Design

All these years later, just knowing he is alive and well provides a thrill. Dr. Tullio Simoncini would have said this is impossible, for he believes that even his expensive treatment with IVs would not do the job of reaching sufficient therapeutic power down to the deep level of bones. He was wrong and that is why I call for universal oral use in all cancers coupled with intensive transdermal applications. Dr. Simoncini does endorse use of oral bicarbonate for certain cancers.

One has to understand that this is perfectly possible. Traditional medical science is beginning to understand this with the early success of a new class of cancer drugs, raising hope among the world's top cancer specialists. The drugs, still in early testing, work in an entirely new way, by unleashing the immune system to attack cancer cells much as it attacks bacteria. That could be an alternative to often-debilitating chemotherapy.

All I have to say here is that baking soda saved my life! Anyone who doubts me should see me now! I had pancreatic cancer and was given 6 to 8 months to live with no hope... today I am pain free, and living a healthy lifestyle to keep it that way. Mrs. Gerson is wrong . . . dead wrong!! Plus, before I went on the protocol, my BP was 246/116. Today it was 114/68, and I haven't taken any BP medication for 5 months! All I did was follow Vern Johnston's protocol to a T, along with the alkaline diet and breathing.

K W

There was one study in which all five patients had their cancers virtually disappear in just a few weeks. According to the New York Times one of the sickest patients, 58-year-old David Aponte, saw his leukemia disappear in just eight days. One does not have to wait for these new drugs that are still in testing, one can depend on sodium bicarbonate and a list of other medicinals in the Natural Allopathic protocol that give you a fighting chance to knock cancer to the ground.

A doctor friend of mine in South Africa, who routinely uses IVs in her practice, said, "Also I found my patients had side effects from the bicarbonate IVs using Simoncini's protocol, so I give it orally. We get the same effect just administering the agents differently. I found this worked best for the patients I was treating. It so easy to give and does not give any discomfort."

To get a clearer vision of how we should do oral bicarbonate treatments, it is pertinent to read what Dr. Tullio Simoncini says about his IV bicarbonate cancer treatment. "Sodium bicarbonate therapy is harmless, fast, and effective because it is extremely diffusible. A therapy with bicarbonate for cancer should be set up with strong dosage, continuously, and with pauseless cycles in a destruction work which should proceed from the beginning to the end without interruption for at least 7 to 8 days. In general a mass of 2 to 3 to 4 centimeters will begin to consistently regress from the third to the fourth day and collapses from the fourth to the fifth," says Simoncini.

Naturopath Parhatsathid Nabadalung says, "The best time to take it is whenever your pH is most acidic, which is during the night. It is best used when pH is around 5.6 to 5.9 (urinary). However, if the pH is below that, then somewhat stronger alkalinity is needed. In which case, I turn to potassium carbonate, potassium bicarbonate and sodium bicarbonate mixture. So if you take these, then both your salivary and urinary pH optimum should align close to each other. The usual dosage for me is $1/_2$ teaspoon (of potassium bicarbonate), $1/_2$ to 1 teaspoon of sodium bicarbonate (now if my pH is very acid, I add $1/_8$ teaspoon of potassium carbonate)."

Bill Henderson, author of *Cancer-Free, Your Guide to Gentle, Non-toxic Healing* mixes 3 parts Grade B maple syrup with one part baking soda and heats the mixture for a couple of minutes on the stove at low temperature. As soon as the baking soda foams up, he takes it off. He keeps it in the fridge and twice a day stirs it up (it settles) and takes one teaspoon. Result: normal and easy bowel movements, twice a day—sometimes three.

Serious Dosages

If you intend to cure yourself of cancer or any serious disease with bicarbonate, you need to plan very carefully the dosages. Dosages need to be strictly adhered too because too much baking soda can cause alkalosis, a blood pH that is too high. Also, and even more importantly, taking too little bicarbonate will not accomplish the mission. So take your urinary and saliva pH every day and sometimes, in the middle of intense bicarbonate therapy, take it many times a day.

One suggested plan for an adult could be a dosage of taking 1 teaspoon in a full glassful of water (instead of half tea in 4 ounces) following that glass of water with another glass of water. A person can do this 3 times a day the first week, 2 times a day the second week, and once a day the third week. The person who followed this routine is doing it once or twice a month to maintain the benefits.

Many find that concentration level too much for oral comfort and for those I suggest much lower concentrations, but then compensate with high concentrated sodium bicarbonate baths with magnesium salts. Soon there will be a product on the market from Japan that will dissolve the sodium bicarbonate into CO_2 micro bubbles in the bath for super absorption.

Vernon Johnston was a pioneer, and his story is important for every cancer patient to read.

My first PSA test registered 22.3, and my doctors made appointments for a biopsy. The biopsy report indicated that I did indeed have prostate cancer. This called for the next step—a bone scan. The report from this scan, as well as a Pelvic Cat Scan, is where the doctors decided I was afflicted with aggressive prostate cancer, dated March 17, 2008: "Reviewed CT and bone scan. Bone scan showed metastatic disease at R sacrum and L illiac wing". So they patted me on the back and told me I had aggressive prostate cancer that had spread to the bone.

A second opinion from another oncologist gave me this report: "Ancillary Studies: These are largely mentioned in the history of present illness. The pathology confirms the presence of prostate carcinoma of high grade. The T stage would appear to be stage III, but without obvious invasion into the seminal vesicles on CT scan. The radionuclide bone scan and plain films confirm the presence of skeletal metastasis in the sacrum and the left illium. In addition, on my review of the CT scan of the pelvis, a number of other small sclerotic lesions are noted within the pelvis. Pre-treatment PSA was 22, but has decreased to 5.88 after institution of Finasteride and Casodex. TNM classification, T#NXM1. AJCC stage IV."

He went on to discuss possible and improbable treatments. What he basically said is that there are none. In fact, he mentioned that he even found a few more spots that the first team of doctors missed.

I was becoming used to the fact that I was a walking dead man. I was anxious to try cesium chloride treatments, but my order got lost in the mail. That is when I decided to do Baking Soda Therapy except that I decided to add Black Strap Molasses as the carrier. I started June 2, 2008 and quit June 12, 2008. I quit because I was scheduled for another bone scan on June 13, 2008. On the way to this test I was hoping for hope. I don't know why I was hoping, because all my research indicated that once cancer got into the bones you are toast. Anyway, I got bone scanned and waited for the report. The report arrived in the mail a few days later. I was nervous and did not want to open it. As a matter of fact, I am crying right now just thinking about it. I finally opened it to these words: "No convincing evidence of an Osseous Metastatic Process." I bawled like a baby.

Two days later, I got another report in the mail about my blood tests: PSA is now 0.1. . . . That is zero point one! My son, by turning me onto adjusting the body's pH from acidic to alkaline as a possible way to create some hope, was a good hit. Arm & Hammer to the rescue! I later found out that Arm & Hammer is shunned by some baking soda users because of the idea that it has aluminum in it. Well, at the time, I could have cared less. As I later found out from research and a visit to a natural food store, aluminum is not in baking soda, it is in baking powder. The employee specializing in the vitamin and mineral department said that Bob's Red Mill Baking Powder is aluminum free and so is, as far as she knew, all baking soda brands.

I am sure many people are interested to know what proportions of baking soda I used with the molasses.

Day One—Day Four : I started out with 1 teaspoon of baking soda with 1 teaspoon of Black Strap molasses and one cup of water. Not warmed or heated water, just room temperature. Next day, the same thing, and that continued through the third and fourth day. My pH measured 7.0 on the fourth day when I did a saliva pH test, and 7.5 when I did a urine pH test. I was feeling fine and decided to up the dose.

Day Five: I started taking the solution twice a day. I also started taking better notes and finally got some pH paper and sticks, so I could measure my pH. My goal was to get to 8.0 to 8.5 pH and hold it for 4 to five days. I read that cancer cells become dormant at pH 7.0 and 7.5 and kills them dead at 8.0 and 8.5. That was my goal. To kill them dead and hoping that bone cancer was a willing victim.

Day Six: I was still taking 2 teaspoons of baking soda with 2 teaspoon of molasses and 1 cup of water twice a day. The pH measured 7.25. Am I getting symptoms? Yes. I am feeling a little nauseous. Not much, but a little queasy. My stool had a yellowish tinge. Now on this day six I really started tracking. I am checking pH with Stix and regular paper pH strips.

(I discovered that all pH papers are not alike.) I test saliva and the urine, but did not track which one at the time.

Here are the times and dosages:

(BSMBS2 refers to a mix of Black Strap Molasses and Baking Soda—2 teaspoons each, and adding water.)

0645—Stix pH 7.25 and 7.75; Paper 7.5 Pee. Stix 7.5 and 6.75 Saliva

1400—BSMBS2

1600—(Stix pH 7.125 Saliva) (Stix pH 7.75 Pee)

2030—BSMBS2

2345—(Stix pH 8.0)—Felt a little nausea

Day Seven: 06/08 1200 (Stix pH 7.375 Paper pH 7.5+) I was getting excited. My lips tingle a bit, and I feel the beginning of Oxygen Euphoria. I was worried a little about the lips, but then recall that some people report this as being part of the cesium therapy. Now the Oxygenation feeling, that is really something else. It felt like I was hooked up to a pure oxygen machine, and my nostrils were as big as wheel barrows. On day seven I got aggressive and increased the baking soda dosage to 3 teaspoons. This brought on a slight headachy feeling. I backed off to 2 teaspoons baking soda because I was getting a little nervous. Also, my headache was getting stronger. I vacillated between continuing with the higher dose or not. I really wanted to kill it. But I went with my feeling and reduced it.

1205—BSM1BS3 Increased BS dosage to 3 teaspoons for this session

1800—(Stix pH 7.75) BSMBS2 got a little nervous about 3 teaspoons, so I backed off to 2 teaspooons

Day Eight: I moved to doing the double dose three times a day. I wanted that pH to get up there.

06/09 0600—(Stix pH 7.7

1000—BSMBS2

1900—(Stix pH 8.25)

1905—BSMBS2

2345—BSMBS2

Day Nine: A little diarrhea, but not much. I am feeling a little weak, but again, not much. Later as I thought back, it would have been a good idea to up my potassium intake.

06/10—0800—pH 7.75

0900—pH 8.25

0905—BSMBS2

1400—pH 8.5 A note: a little diarrhea, but not much

1600—BSMBS2

1730—pH 8.75

2200—pH 8.5

2345—BSMBS2 A note: Felt oxygenation euphoria throughout the day. Like my body was breathing pure oxygen. Nostrils are at least a mile wide.

Day Ten: My headache is more persistent, and I am having body sweats at night. Again, I experienced the sweats, duplicating cesium symptoms. I cut back this day to a solution twice a day, not three times.

06/11 0800—pH 8.5

0830—BSMBS2

1230—pH 8.5

1830—pH 8.5 Headache

2330—8.375

2331—BSMBS2 Note: Headache most of the day and part of yesterday. Felt sweaty late at night. Cut back to BSMBS2 only twice today.

Day Eleven: My last day before I am scheduled for the big test. The body scan, that is, to check on the condition of my bones, to see what is going on with the cancer.

06/12 0800—(pH 8.0 and 7.5) Going down to 2 times a day

0910—pH 7.25

0920—BSMBS1.5 Note: Dropped to 1.5 teaspoons to see if it would help control headache. Experienced a loose stool and slight headache, felt sweaty last night.

1020—More diarrhea with slight yellow tinge. Note: Cutting back because I felt like it. I felt like I was getting overloaded. I probably would not have dropped back if I was not going to have body scan at hospital tomorrow.

1300—pH 8.35

Important Notes on pH Readings

What ph level should we get the urine or saliva up to? Your ph can go too high, which also invites certain illnesses and imbalances in the body, and this is the purpose of the monitoring with the pH paper—to keep pH in a healthy range.

> *When you take your saliva pH, take it at least one hour before or 2 hours after you eat. Take measurements 2 to 3 times a day, so you can get a feel for what your average is.*

A pH levels in your saliva can be affected by bacteria in your mouth, as well as food you recently ate. In a perfect world with all other health parameters in place, the "averaged" pH of both urine and saliva will be right around what? That's a good question and is best answered perhaps not by a pH strip, but by ones optimum feelings and state of being. Some people think that a pH as low as 6.4 is a good urinary target, but there are some large assumptions that can put us into doubt about this. Getting this one right is important because oxygen levels in the body are directly related to pH levels. Increasing pH from 4 pH to 5 pH increases oxygen to the cells by ten-fold, from a 4 pH to a 6 pH increases oxygen by 100 times, and raising pH from 4 pH to 7 pH increases oxygen levels by 1,000 times.

> *When body pH drops below 6.4, enzymes are deactivated, digestion does not work properly; vitamins, minerals and food supplements cannot effectively assimilate.*

Understand that pH can move all over the place.[2] This is so because most individual's "total alkalinity" is not very strong, and that is exactly what bicarbonate therapy, as well as, exercise, dietary sanity, and good breathing promote, total alkalinity. So, for instance, two hours after a meal you may find the urine going acid, as it is a reflection of the meals acid components pushing the pH. With life threatening situations we don't want to be eating meals with large acid components, so our urinary drift into the acidic with meals can be very mild if one is eating and fasting correctly.

We should not be surprised or disturbed when we see urinary pH getting down into the 5 range sometimes, as this is a reflection of kidney capacity and it shows metabolic acids can and are being removed from the system. You want your urine to be able to move acid, and to essentially be acidic when appropriate. For cancer treatment, we want to break past this and establish a pH of around 8 for two weeks and then take a break letting urinary pH fall.

16. *Sodium Bicarbonate Baths*

Sodium bicarbonate baths are an excellent way of increasing bicarbonate levels in the body. Athletes will appreciate taking such baths. The theory behind loading up on bicarbonates before sports performances is that by neutralizing the acid (lactic) produced by muscle cells during anaerobic exercise, the pH level of the working muscle will be kept in an optimal range for peak performance considerably longer.

Scientific Findings

A study done in 1993 looked at the effect of sodium bicarbonate ingestion (300mg/kg body weight) on isokinetic leg extension/flexion exercises. The exercise consisted of leg extension/flexion with the first set consisting of four reps at a speed of 60 degrees/second. Consequently, the second set consisted of 60 reps at a speed of 240 degrees/second; this set lasted about 85 seconds. More work was performed by subjects using sodium bicarbonate when compared to the placebo/control conditions. When workload was increased to above 80 percent of maximal oxygen uptake, which makes it partly anaerobic for most people, the perceived effort was less when bicarbonate was taken, indicating that the perceived workload was less strenuous. Dr D Wilkes at York University, Toronto, reported a 2.9 seconds faster running time over a distance of 800 meters using 300mg/kg bodyweight of sodium bicarbonate.[1] The 2.9 seconds average improvement translates to a distance of 19 meters. In an 800 meter race, that's a huge difference.

Dr David Costill and colleagues at the Human Performance Laboratory at Ball State University, Indiana gave their athletes 200 mg/kg bodyweight of sodium bicarbonate The athletes then did five, one minute sprints on an ergometer bicycle, the last one to absolute exhaustion. The baking soda loading improved the time to exhaustion of the last sprint by an incredible 42 percent.[2] Other studies[3] have also reported increased endurance, and increased power output after soda loading in maximal short term exercise.

Dr. GW Mainwood and colleagues in 1980 discovered that the less acidic blood becomes when filled with bicarbonate, the more it creates what is called a pH gradient between muscle and blood, which pulls acid out of the muscle.[4] Athletes who rely heavily on the use of the lactic acid energy system during exercise, such as bodybuilders, get the most benefits from alkaline salts, in contrast to endurance athletes who find them not beneficial since purely aerobic athletic events do not produce lactate rapidly in the muscle cell.

Over a period of 50 years, research conducted in the USA and Germany relating to alkaline salts revealed significant physiological improvement with anaerobic exercise, treadmill, and bicycle ergometer exercise tests to exhaustion. Other studies have revealed no significant improvements in these areas, but generally they have used lower doses of bicarbonate or have used exercise duration greater than 5 minutes.[5]

A fairly recent study[6], done in Australia at the Tasmanian Institute of Technology, gave elite class rowers 300 mg/kg bodyweight of bicarbonate or placebo. Ninety-five minutes later, subjects made a maximal effort for six minutes on a rowing ergometer. Compared with placebo, the subjects rowed almost 50 meters further in the same time when receiving sodium bicarbonate.

Transdermal Use

Sodium bicarbonate can provide a winning edge, especially for sports demanding all out effort for periods of about 30 seconds to six minutes, although the lactic acid energy system may also be involved in activities of lesser and greater time periods than this range.

There is one big problem for athletes when ingesting sodium bicarbonate. Many of the subjects in the research studies experienced some form of gastro intestinal distress, about 60 minutes after ingesting the bicarbonate solution. This includes belching and diarrhea. One investigator noted that several of his subjects had what he termed "explosive diarrhea." Such conditions could be debilitating to athletic performance.

One way that has been suggested to avoid this is by taking bicarbonate every 20 minutes in divided doses, beginning three hours before the event and ending one hour before the start. The second way would be to take a strong bicarbonate bath with one to several pounds of baking soda mixed with some Dead Sea salt or pure magnesium chloride. I would lowball the magnesium part of such a bath before events because of its relaxing effect, but one could jump in and out of a very strong bicarbonate bath and avoid the complications baking soda causes in some gastrointestinal systems.

An adequate oral dose would be about 300 mg per kg of body weight mixed with around 400 ml of liquid, for example a 90 kg bodybuilder would take 27 grams on an empty stomach approximately 30 to 60 minutes before exercise. The bi-carb can be mixed with water or other beverages.

When magnesium salts and baking soda are combined in the bath, the combination may reduce the negative effects of minor exposure to the radiation from X-rays.

Adding a cup or two of baking soda to a hot bath after a long exhausting day alleviates tension and muscle aches. It exfoliates the skin to remove dead dry skin, leaving fresh bright youthful skin behind without the high cost of the commercial skin exfoliates. Adding baking soda to foot baths help with tired, achy feet when working in jobs, such as waitressing or other heavy-walking-type jobs.

Combining the baking soda with magnesium salts brings dramatic changes to human physiology, and the only thing making this formula even better would be the addition of some sodium thiosulfate (neutralizes chlorine) for a full hot springs therapeutic treatment.

To assess statistically the efficacy of sodium bicarbonate baths in psoriasis patients, thirty-one with mild-moderate psoriasis were studied. Almost all patients who used $NaHCO_3^-$ reported a statistically valuable improvement. $NaHCO_3^-$ baths reduced itchiness and irritation; in general, the patients themselves recognized a beneficial impact on their psoriasis, so much so that they have continued to bathe in $NaHCO_3$ even after the end of the study.[7] When patients combine this with transdermal magnesium therapy, they will have a clear resolution of psoriasis.

17. Warnings and Contraindications

Everything needs to be taken in balance. Sodium bicarbonate (baking soda) is generally well tolerated. However, high doses may cause headache, nausea, or irritability. If any of these effects continue or become bothersome, inform your doctor. Notify your doctor if you develop: muscle weakness, slow reflexes and confusion, swelling of the feet or ankles, black tar-like stools, coffee-ground vomit. If you notice other effects not listed above, contact your doctor or pharmacist.

Dr. Mark Pagel said, "Baking soda is not necessarily safe. It is known from pre-clinical studies and mathematical oncology modeling that too much baking soda, and/or baking soda treatment that is continued for too long, will be harmful to normal tissues, especially kidney and bladder tissues. The problem is that the level that is "too much" and the time that is "too long" is unknown, and probably differs for different people (for example, older patients with limited kidney function are likely more sensitive to baking soda treatment). Therefore, there is a real concern that too much baking soda applied for too long may harm a patient.

Safe Use

The key to safe use of sodium bicarbonate is the monitoring and testing of both urinary and saliva pH with pH test paper or an electronic tester. I recommend people do this every morning and chart their results, and whenever taking strong baking soda baths, do the same thing soon after getting out of the tub. We do not want the urinary pH to go over 8.0, and Arm & Hammer suggests right on the box to stop therapy, to let the pH drop back down after a week of high use.

One can overdo anything! When I say baking soda is safe, I mean it is exceptionally safe if you compare it with overly strong poisons found in chemotherapies. Sodium bicarbonate is a strong medicinal, one of the strongest, and it will drive pH levels up quickly throughout most of the tissues, and that is why it is so effective.

Do not use if you are on a sodium restricted diet unless directed by a doctor. Ask a doctor or a pharmacist before use if you are taking a prescription drug. Antacids may interact with certain prescription drugs. Do not administer to children under age 5 without careful consideration. To avoid injury, do not take sodium bicarbonate until the powder is completely dissolved and it is very important not to take baking soda when overly full from food or drink. Consult a doctor if severe stomach pain occurs after taking this product. "I nearly died after taking this stuff," said William Graves, who suffered a rupture through the wall of his stomach in 1979 after taking baking soda mixed in water for indigestion after a big meal. The 64-year-old resident of Bethesda, Maryland, who is editor of *National Geographic Magazine*, said that only emergency surgery saved his life and that six more operations were needed to repair the damage. Though there are only a few documented cases, users need to know of the dangers.

The aim of all bicarbonate therapy is to produce a substantial correction of the low total CO_2 content and blood pH, but the risks of over dosage and alkalosis should be avoided. In general, dose selection for pregnant women, young infants, and elderly patients should be cautious, usually starting at the low end of the dosing range, reflecting the greater frequency of decreased hepatic, renal, or cardiac function and of concomitant disease or other drug therapy.

Adverse Reactions:

- Overly aggressive therapy with Sodium Bicarbonate Injection, USP can result in metabolic alkalosis (associated with muscular twitchings, irritability, and tetany) and hypernatremia. Caution should also be maintained when pushing oral dosages up to the maximum levels suggested for oral administration as well.

Overdosage:

- Should alkalosis result, the bicarbonate should be stopped and the patient managed according to the degree of alkalosis present. Ninetenths percent sodium chloride injection intravenous may be given; potassium chloride also may be indicated if there is hypokalemia. Severe alkalosis may be accompanied by hyperirritability or tetany and these symptoms may be controlled by calcium gluconate.

Contraindications

For people with the rare illnesses of Bartter syndrome or Gitelman syndrome, bicarbonate may be contraindicated. These rare sufferers may add a few drops of Real-Lemon juice concentrate to any bicarbonate-containing beverage to neutralize it.

Serious precautions should be taken by individuals who suffer from chronic pulmonary problems. If a person has significant lung disease, their brain shifts to breathing in response to a lowered O_2 level so it won't respond to the accumulating CO_2. With the added CO_2 and the lungs not removing it, the equation shifts left, meaning the added CO_2 becomes $H2CO_3$ (carbonic acid) and then you end up with an acidic patient

Sodium Bicarbonate Injection, USP is contraindicated in patients who are losing chloride by vomiting or from continuous gastrointestinal suction, and in patients receiving diuretics known to produce a hypochloremic alkalosis.

Solutions containing sodium ions should be used with great care, if at all, in patients with congestive heart failure, severe renal insufficiency, and in clinical states in which there exists edema with sodium retention. In patients with diminished renal function, administration of solutions containing sodium ions may result in sodium retention. The intravenous administration of these solutions can cause fluid and/or solute overloading resulting in dilution of serum electrolyte concentrations, overhydration, congested states, or pulmonary edema. *Extra caution* needs to be taken with cancer patients with severe heart, renal, and hepatic problems.

Adverse reactions to the administration of sodium bicarbonate can include metabolic alkalosis, edema due to sodium overload, congestive heart failure, hyperosmolar syndrome, hypervolemic hypernatremia, and hypertension due to increased sodium. In patients who consume high calcium or dairy-rich diet, calcium supplements, or calcium-containing antacids, such as calcium carbonate (for example, Tums), the use of sodium bicarbonate can cause milk-alkali syndrome, which can result in metastatic calcification, kidney stones, and kidney failure. In rare cases, metabolic alkalosis develops in a person who has ingested too much base from substances, such as baking soda (bicarbonate of soda). Severe metabolic alkalosis (for example, blood pH >7.55) is a serious medical problem. Mortality rates have been reported as 45 percent in patients with an arterial blood pH of 7.55 and 80 percent when the pH was greater than 7.65.

Administration of sodium bicarbonate in amounts that exceed the capacity of the kidneys to excrete this excess bicarbonate may cause metabolic alkalosis. This capacity is reduced when a reduction in filtered bicarbonate occurs, as observed in renal failure, or when enhanced tubular reabsorption of bicarbonate occurs, as observed in volume depletion.[1]

Metabolic alkalosis is the most common acid-base disturbance observed in hospitalized patients, accounting for approximately 50 percent of all acid-base disorders.

- Severe alkalosis causes diffuse arteriolar constriction with reduction in tissue perfusion. By decreasing cerebral blood flow, alkalosis may lead to tetany, seizures, and decreased mental status. Metabolic alkalosis also decreases coronary blood flow and predisposes persons to refractory arrhythmias.

- Metabolic alkalosis causes hypoventilation, which may cause hypoxemia, especially in patients with poor respiratory reserve, and it may impair weaning from mechanical ventilation.

- Alkalosis decreases the serum concentration of ionized calcium by increasing calcium ion binding to albumin. In addition, metabolic alkalosis is almost always associated with hypokalemia (low potassium levels), which can cause neuromuscular weakness and arrhythmias, and, by increasing ammonia production, it can precipitate hepatic encephalopathy in susceptible individuals.

The physical signs of metabolic alkalosis are not specific and depend on the severity of the alkalosis. Because metabolic alkalosis decreases ionized calcium concentration, signs of hypocalcemia (for example, tetany, Chvostek sign, Trousseau sign), change in mental status or seizures may be present.

Symptoms of Alkalosis:

- Confusion(can progress to stupor or coma)

- Hand tremor

- Light-headedness

- Muscle twitching

- Nausea, vomiting

- Numbness or tingling in the face or extremities

- Prolonged muscle spasms (tetany)

Tell your doctor if you have: pre-existing heart disease, kidney disease, liver disease, high blood pressure, or any allergies. Because this medication contains a large amount of sodium, remind your doctor if you are on a low sodium diet. This medication should be used only if clearly needed during pregnancy. Small amounts of sodium bicarbonate have been found to be present in breast milk. Discuss the risks and benefits with your doctor even though he or she probably may not be fully aware of the benefits.

Tell your doctor of any over-the-counter or prescription medication you may take and ask him about dangers and side effects that are common with such drugs. This medication has the potential to interact with many medications. Do not take any other medication within 1 to 2 hours of taking an antacid. If overdose is suspected, contact your local poison control center or emergency room immediately. US residents can call the US national poison hotline at 800-222-1222. Canadian residents should call their local poison control center directly. Symptoms of overdose may include irritability, muscle rigidity, and seizures. Before taking sodium bicarbonate, tell your doctor if you are taking the following:

- mecamylamine (Inversine

- methenamine (Mandelamine)

- ketoconazole (Nizoral)

- antacids

- a tetracycline antibiotic such as tetracycline (Sumycin, Achromycin V, and others), demeclocycline (Declomycin), doxycycline (Vibramycin, Monodox, Doxy, and others), minocycline (Minocin, Dynacin, and others), or oxytetracycline (Terramycin, and others)

You may not be able to take sodium bicarbonate, or you may require a dosage adjustment, or special monitoring during treatment if you are taking any of the medicines listed above. If you miss a dose, take it as soon as remembered; do not take it if it is near the time for the next dose, instead, skip the missed dose and resume your usual dosing schedule. Do not "double-up" the dose to catch up. Store at room temperature, between 59 and 86 degrees F (between 15 and 30 degrees C), away from heat, light, and moisture.

Make sure you only take a small amount of baking soda solution at any given time, since alkaline substances can neutralize most if not all acids in the stomach, causing the stomach to create more acid. This can, in turn, lead to more heartburn, which will cause you to ingest more baking soda solution and start a dangerous cycle. Folic acid is needed by the body to utilize Vitamin B12.[2] Antacids, including sodium bicarbonate, inhibit folic acid absorption.[1] People taking antacids are advised to supplement with folic acid.

It can also be applied topically as a paste, with three parts baking soda to one part water, to relieve insect bites.

Using Sodium Bicarbonate

One should approach using baking soda with a measure of care and respect for the warnings and contraindications, but in reality what we are dealing with is one of the safest medicines. It is useful to know that taking baking soda as an antacid can rupture your stomach if you take it when over full? There have only been a handful of cases during the last hundred years, but it does happen. People who have grossly overeaten and have had a severely distended stomach found that taking baking soda as an antacid can indeed generate enough carbon dioxide to rupture the stomach.

18. *Magnesium Bicarbonate*

Magnesium bicarbonate is a complex hydrated salt that exists only in water under specific conditions. There are, however, a few companies that sell magnesium bicarbonate water, instead we have a magnesium bicarbonate concentrate. Magnesium and bicarbonate rich mineral waters are easily absorbed and have many health benefits. The magnesium ion is Mg_2^+ and the bicarbonate ion is HCO_3^-. So, magnesium bicarbonate must have two bicarbonate ions: $Mg(HCO_3)_2$. Magnesium bicarbonate is the *Ultimate Mitochondrial Cocktail*. In the presence of magnesium and bicarbonate ions, less acid is produced by carbonic anhydrase enzyme.[1]

Uses

Low serum and intracellular magnesium concentrations are associated with insulin resistance, impaired glucose tolerance, and decreased insulin secretion.[2,3,4] We need large amounts of magnesium and bicarbonate ions for smooth running physiology. Alkalosis enhances magnesium reabsorption in the juxtamedullary proximal nephron.[5] It is magnesium that modulates cellular events involved in inflammation. Magnesium literally puts the chill on inflammation. Magnesium deficiencies feed the fires of inflammation and pain. Sodium bicarbonate does the same, so when used together we can expect exponentially better results.

Magnesium bicarbonate buffers the mitochondria in body cells from excess acid concentrations, which improves mitochondrial function and allows more ATP to be produced. Magnesium bicarbonate protects the natural organic and inorganic phosphate buffers in the cytoplasm of cells. Magnesium bicarbonate neutralizes the acid produced as a result of metabolic processes and ATP hydrolysis. This allows more ATP to be hydrolyzed; that is, more energy can be utilized. The kidneys represent the water element in

Chinese medicine, and the most effective method of regulating its health and function is with these water elements, magnesium chloride and sodium bicarbonate, both of which are heavily present in the sea and in all good mineral waters.

Bicarbonate ion concentrations decrease the formation of acid by carbonic anhydrase enzyme (Le Chatelier's principle). In the presence of magnesium and bicarbonate ions, less acid is produced by carbonic anhydrase enzyme.[6] Sodium bicarbonate-rich mineral water, in conjunction with a low-salt diet, has a beneficial effect on calcium homeostasis.[7]

Few clinicians are aware how these two substances work to enhance each other—they are mutually reinforcing because magnesium functions as a bicarbonate co-transporter into cells, and *bicarbonate acts as a transporter of magnesium into the mitochondria.* Magnesium influx is linked with bicarbonate transport according to the *Dietary Reference Intakes* guide from the Institute of Medicine. Magnesium transport into or out of cells requires the presence of carrier-mediated transport systems (Gunther, 1003; Romani et al., 1993).[8]

ATPase reaction has a broad pH optimum centering on neutral pH, with little significant activity above pH9.0 or below pH5.5.[9] Thus, anything that moves us from overall acid conditions toward alkaline that recover the neutral zone is going to enhance cell metabolism via mitochondrial optimization.

Alkalosis enhances magnesium reabsorption in the juxtamedullary proximal nephron.[10]It was the dedicated work of Dr. Russell Beckett, a veterinarian with a PhD in biochemical pathology that paved the way to understand the significance of bicarbonate acting in conjunction with magnesium. He has formulated *Unique Water* which, it has been asserted, slowed the aging process and increased the length of life of humans and other mammals and could be used to treat all inflammatory and degenerative diseases. *Unique Water* is water containing magnesium bicarbonate. Dr. Beckett's research has resulted in the understanding how important both bicarbonate and magnesium ions are in human physiology, and how they work together to optimize human health and the ability to recover from disease.

Bicarbonate ions working alongside magnesium would naturally create the conditions for increased glucose transport across cell plasma membranes. Bicarbonate ions without doubt create the alkaline conditions for maintaining the enzyme activity of pancreatic secretions in the intestines. Bicarbonate neutralize acid conditions required for inflammatory reactions. Hence, sodium bicarbonate would be of benefit in the treatment of a range of chronic inflammatory and autoimmune diseases.

Bicarbonate acts to stimulate the ATPase by acting directly on it.[11] Magnesium does not readily reach the mitochondrion, but if plenty of bicarbonate is available, the bicarbonate will act as transport into the mitochondrion. The only problem is that the few magnesium bicarbonate products available for sale are expensive compared to using magnesium chloride and sodium bicarbonate individually. It is possible though, that one can always make their own magnesium bicarbonate.[12]

Carbonic anhydrase (CA) is a ubiquitous metalloenzyme that catalyzes the reversible hydration/dehydration of carbon dioxide. Carbonic anhydrase enzyme is ever-present in body cells and constitutes up to 10 percent of the soluble protein in most body cells. It is one of the fastest enzymes known: each carbonic anhydrase enzyme produces from ten thousand to one million acid groups (H+) per second. The acid (H+) produced by carbonic anhydrase enzyme is pumped by proton pump enzymes into cell organelles, such as lysosomes, phagosomes, endosomes, and ruffled membranes. In red blood cells (rbcs), CA is the second most abundant protein to hemoglobin and plays a crucial role in CO_2 transport. More specifically, rbc CA catalyzes the hydration of CO_2 to HCO_3^- at the tissue site of production and the dehydration of HCO -3 to CO_2 at the respiratory surface, thereby facilitating the transport and excretion of CO_2 from the body.[13] In addition, rbc CA also facilitates the linkage of O_2 and CO_2 transport via the Bohr effect.[14] Carbonic anhydrase speeds the reaction of carbon dioxide and water. This reaction produces carbonic acid, which quickly dissociates into bicarbonate and hydrogen ions.

Bicarbonate ion concentrations decrease the formation of acid by carbonic anhydrase enzyme (Le Chatelier's principle). In the presence of magnesium and bicarbonate ions, less acid is produced by carbonic anhydrase enzyme.[15] But studies with partially purified carbonic anhydrase from spinach (Spinaciaoleracea L.) chloroplasts show that the effect was the result of the chloride ion and not the magnesium ion. Enzyme activity was reduced 50 percent upon addition of 3 to 10 millimolar $MgCl_2$ or KCl, while all additions of $MgSO_4$ between 0.3 and 10 millimolar were mildly stimulatory.[16]

Excess acid accumulation leads to oxygen deprivation and thus, cell fermentation. Acid conditions lead to cell rot, another term for cancer. Magnesium stabilizes ATP[17], allowing DNA and RNA transcriptions and repairs.[18] Higher pH levels and the bicarbonate itself will help the magnesium leave the blood serum, driving Mg_2^+ into the cells where again the bicarbonate will carry it from the cytoplasm into the mitochondria where, in cases of chronic disease, it is desperately needed. Thus magnesium and bicarbonate, when used together, would considerably increase the energy production in body cells.

> *Mg2+ is critical for all of the energetics of the cells because it is absolutely required that Mg$_2$+ be bound by ATP, the central high energy compound of the body.*
> —Dr. Boyd Haley

Magnesium bicarbonate decreases the production of acid from carbon dioxide in body cells. Magnesium and bicarbonate would at the same time increase energy in several ways. First, magnesium bicarbonate *protects* the natural organic and inorganic phosphate buffers in the cytoplasm of cells. Second, magnesium bicarbonate *neutralizes* the acid produced as a result of metabolic processes and ATP hydrolysis. This allows more ATP to be hydrolyzed; that is, more energy can be utilized. Magnesium bicarbonate *buffers* the mitochondria in body cells from excess acid concentrations, which improves mitochondrial function and allows more ATP to be produced. When more ATP can be hydrolyzed and more ATP can be produced, body cells have sufficient energy for optimum function.

> *ATP without Mg2+ bound cannot create the energy normally used by specific enzymes of the body to make protein, DNA, RNA, transport sodium or potassium or calcium in and out of cells. ATP without enough Mg2+ is non-functional and leads to cell death.*
> —Dr. Boyd Haley

Dr. Seeger and Dr. Budwig, in Germany, have shown that cancer is mainly the result of a faulty energy metabolism in the powerhouses of the cells—the mitochondria. ATP and most of the enzymes involved in the production of energy require magnesium. A healthy cell has high magnesium and low calcium levels. The problem that comes with low magnesium (Mg) levels is the calcium builds up inside the cells while energy production decreases as the mitochondria gradually calcify.

Magnesium ions constitute the physiologically active magnesium in the body; they are not attached to other substances and are free to join in biochemical body processes.[19]Bicarbonate ions neutralize carbonic acid formed in the body during metabolic processes. Several studies have shown that an increased intake of bicarbonate may help prevent muscle wasting and bone loss. Our diets are usually acidic. Acids burn out our cells and causes accelerated aging. Bicarbonate is alkaline and provides the body with the extra alkalinity needed by the body to neutralize excess acidity.

Magnesium is often lost in urine as a consequence of too much acid in the body. If your urine is too acidic, it indicates you are losing magnesium. Alkaline water with magnesium, bicarbonate, calcium, and potassium increases pH significantly. Bicarbonate alkaline mineral water can increase urinary volume, pH, citrate, uric acid, and magnesium excretion of renal stone forming objects by consumption of at least 2lit/day.[20]

The most important effect of bicarbonate ingestion is the change in acid-base balance, as well as blood pH and bicarbonate concentration in biological fluids. This is especially important and useful medically when you consider the fact that normal adult humans eating typical American diets characteristically have chronic, low-grade metabolic acidosis.[21] When it comes to acid alkaline balance, we are what we eat and doctors have to face the reality of the huge mistake our civilization and our patients make in this regard.

Dosages

Magnesium bicarbonate is like drinking water from a fountain of youth and that is exactly how you drink it. $Mg2^+$ in water is highly bioavailable and waterborne $Mg2^+$ is absorbed approximately 30 percent faster and better than $Mg2^+$ from food. Consequently, $Mg2^+$ supplementation may be best achieved using a high $Mg2^+$ nutrient with the best bioavailability, such as drinking water.

One needs to take 56,400 mg of sodium bicarbonate to get 41,800 mg of bicarbonate. But when one takes magnesium bicarbonate, one gets no sodium and all the magnesium and bicarbonate reaches into the cells helping each other pass through the cell walls. When you take magnesium bicarbonate you get super high dosages of bicarbonate because there are two bicarbonate ions to each magnesium ion.

In my *Water Medicine* book you will find out that drinking water with magnesium bicarbonate will extend your life, ease your pains, and make your children stronger. It is the fountain of youth, and those who drink enough of such waters at the right concentrations will find the promised gift. There is an intense therapeutic effect when one doses with large dosages of magnesium that just does not happen at lower therapeutic dosages. Same goes for bicarbonate. Some emergency room and intensive care doctors will understand immediately what I am talking about and so will any doctor who uses intravenous magnesium administration. With the new magnesium bicarbonate concentrate, one can take their magnesium and bicarbonate intake up to very high therapeutic dosages, and that is going to make a world of difference for people in dire medical need.

19. *Sodium and Magnesium Bicarbonate Products*

Though I have been using Bob's Red Mill sodium bicarbonate, I have recently received two boxes of Arm & Hammer, and I sat for quite a while admiring their boxes and all the information on them. I have been in touch directly with the company and have been reassured of its absolute purity, meaning there is no aluminum in it. Arm & Hammer is as aluminum free as Bob's Red Mill, which advertises itself specifically to be aluminum free and in the process has convinced most people I know that Arm & Hammer has aluminum, when it does not.

Sodium Bicarbonate

Many have determined that the sodium bicarbonate contained in 8-ounce boxes of Arm & Hammer Baking Soda® was sufficiently constant in weight that dissolved in water to a given volume, it yielded a quantitatively acceptable therapeutic solution of sodium bicarbonate at an incredibly low cost. Grocery store baking soda is a safe, economical, and convenient source of sodium bicarbonate for the treatment of chronic metabolic acidosis in infants and young children.[1]

The Church & Dwight name may not be familiar to many people, but their Arm & Hammer® brand is recognized and respected by just about everyone. That's because Church & Dwight has been producing Arm & Hammer brand products for almost 160 years, ever since Austin Church, a physician, and John Dwight, his brother-in-law, began selling their high-quality sodium bicarbonate to grocers in New York City.

The most demanding applications are in the area of healthcare, with hemodialysis, in particular, requiring exceptional purity and consistency. A leading force in modern bicarbonate hemodialysis, Church & Dwight's contribution to modern dialysis dates back to the early 1980s, when medical literature about the benefits of bicarbonate-buffered dialysate over acetate began to appear.

Bob's Red Mill costs $2.61 a pound and Arm & Hammer costs less, making it the least expensive medicine in the world. Personally, I could not tell a difference between the consistencies in the two, both are equally fine. Sodium bicarbonate is widely available in most supermarkets and discount chains across the country at a cost of just over $2 per pound. One can also buy it for much less in fifty pound sizes.

Do not confuse baking soda with *baking powder*, which does or may contain aluminum. These are two very different products, with *baking powder* having a mix of baking soda with various acidic ingredients. Make sure you are purchasing pure 100 percent baking soda or sodium bicarbonate.

Magnesium Bicarbonate

For years I have searched for a product that combines the best of magnesium and bicarbonate, without the potential side effects of too much chloride and sodium, as is possible when using sodium bicarbonate and magnesium chloride. I have written about the mysterious and hard to come by magnesium bicarbonate as the Ultimate Mitochondria Cocktail. Nothing will do more to overcome mitochondrial decay and general low levels of cell energy than jacking in high levels of magnesium bicarbonate into the cells. Magnesium bicarbonate occurs in nature as rare mountain spring water with a concentration of around 400 parts per million and very little calcium in it. However, my magnesium bicarbonate has 50,000 PPM (5 percent by weight) of magnesium bicarbonate, this elusive compound does not exist in the solid state, so that it is not possible to process it into a pill. Further, it is easy to dilute the concentrate down to 1500 PPM (4 ounces of concentrate into a gallon of calcium-free water) making this the ultimate best healing curative water in the world. Magnesium bicarbonate will help the soft tissues recover their original ability to process healthy nutrition correctly and eliminate wastes.

Sports nutrition has already recognized this, and researchers have found that deep ocean mineral water accelerates *recovery from physical fatigue*. The deep sea is the only place one can actually find magnesium bicarbonate. My water processing system will put out excellent water high in bicarbonates and magnesium for a minimum of cost. The magnesium oil

I recommended for years, that people spread all over their skin (also magnesium gel) and take baths with (flakes), takes care of the transdermal administration of magnesium into the body for often instant anti-inflammatory effect. I have always told cancer patients to get five magnesium massages a week and it is the ultimate 'Cleopatra' type of treatment.

Magnesium bicarbonate though is the Holy Grail of Natural Allopathic Medicine, for it combines my work with sodium bicarbonate with my passion for magnesium medicine. We can consider magnesium bicarbonate to be rocket fuel for the mitochondrial factories inside the cells. The reason I turned so strongly to Transdermal Magnesium Therapy six years ago was because of the limitations of oral magnesium supplementation. That limit has now been resolved allowing for safe and effective oral magnesium intake.

The clear concentrated magnesium bicarbonate solution contains 5 percent by weight of fully reacted magnesium bicarbonate and another total .5 percent of several other mineral bicarbonates, sulfates, and chlorides. The final process wraps all the individual mineral molecules in Buckminster-Fuller cages of hexagonal and pentagonal water clusters, meaning this water will have many layers of water clusters around the magnesium bicarbonate compound.

When we make therapeutic drinking water out of 30 cc of this magnesium bicarbonate product in 1 liter of distilled or other calcium-free water (with a 4 hour waiting period to form the clusters), this water contains 1500 PPM of water-chelated magnesium bicarbonate and another 150PPM of various sea minerals; 1,500 parts per million translates into 1,500 mg/liter of magnesium bicarbonate.

Water made in this way will have around 100 milligrams of glucose per deciliter, which corresponds to around a blood sugar content of 100 on a blood sugar meter. The water has about one calorie per 8 ounce glass, which is barely detectable to the taste, but which makes it very, very desirable to the energy thirsty cells. As it happens, at 1500PPM, one finds that the Activated Magnesium Bicarbonate is actually made of "water balloons" with about one magnesium bicarbonate at the center, one glucose molecule along with it, and 3 to 5 layers of hexagonal bucky-ball layers. The balloons are soft and squishy and the water feels almost "syrupy" on the tongue.

For everyone's convenience I suggest this *bicarbonate formula*, not only because it is easy to take your bicarbonate, but you also get the needed potassium, which is very helpful for cancer patients as it is for everyone else.

Reduced L-Glutathione™ Plus capsules are specially engineered, without excipients, using high purity pharmaceutical grade reduced L-glutathione and sodium bicarbonate. Reduced L-Glutathione™ Plus Capsules can be administered via nebulizer without tissue irritation. An isotonic solution is produced when one Reduced L-Glutathione™ Plus capsule is dissolved in roughly 5 milliliters of distilled water. Cost is $35.00. These capsules are perfect for nebulization. Another excellent way of getting glutathione is through suppositories.

Magnesium Chloride

When it comes to magnesium oil, I recommend only the best, Ancient Minerals. This product is of the absolute highest quality, meaning it can be used for any application, even for eye washes and IV solutions. Coming from a 250 million year old sea deposit below Europe, it is the purest and most powerful medicine in the world. A three month supply of 64 ounces is approximately $100.00.

For magnesium baths there are magnesium chloride bath flakes, as well as Dead Sea and Epsom salts. I rarely recommend oral magnesium pills, preferring transdermal application, and the use of *magnesium oil* for oral use because liquid minerals tend to have much higher absorption rates than solid pill forms. If one is to use intensive therapeutic baths, one could easily use fifty pounds in the three months of intensive protocol application.

Conclusion

Over the last few years, television has been flooded with drug commercials that make it sound as if pharmaceutical companies have discovered the cure for practically every ill . . . that is, until you hear the closing lines of their ads. "Our product is not for everyone." "If rashes, extensive bleeding, and severe headaches occur, stop taking the product, and call your physician immediately." And then there's, "In some rare instances, deaths have occurred." I guess in these last cases, there's no need to call your doc.

The fact is that pharmaceutical companies make billions of dollars in profits each and every year, and they cleverly use their profits to influence government legislators and agencies, the medical community, and the public to believe that their products are the answer to all of our health problems. What they aren't telling us is that, according to a study published in *JAMA*, over 100,000 Americans die each year from *properly* prescribed drugs taken *correctly*. According to the Centers of Disease Control statistics, only 10,000 to 20,000 Americans die annually from taking illegal drugs, so although we have a growing drug problem, it seems that the major culprits are not the drug cartels but the drug companies.

For thousands of years, traditional healers have used natural substances to overcome various illnesses. Through experimentation, trial and error, refinements, and adjustments, many of these natural remedies have been passed down from one generation to another with excellent results—and with few, if any, side effects. Over the last century, drug companies found that many of the most effective natural treatments were inexpensive and unpatentable. This means that no one person or company can own and sell them. But the companies also discovered that by extracting the "active ingredients" and reformulating these natural cures, they could develop patented products. As these companies grew and prospered, the war against natural treatments began—and, to a great degree, it is still underway.

This book has been written to explain the powerful healing properties of sodium bicarbonate. As you have learned, this simple substance can be of great help in combating a host of diseases. It is my hope that this is the first step in your journey back to health. As you move forward in your search for answers, I have no doubt that you will find many contradictory studies and statements. In today's world, it isn't easy to become an informed health advocate for yourself or for another. But if you keep an open mind, learn as much as you can, and determine who's behind the information you are reading, you will be able to slowly uncover the road to greater well-being.

I encourage you to find the answers that are right for you, just as I have. Please feel free to read my blogs at www.greenmedinfo.com. In the meantime, I wish you and yours the best of health.

Resources

NATURAL ALLOPATHIC MEDICINE PROTOCOL COMPONENTS

The Natural Allopathic Medicine protocol is powerful and at the same time extraordinarily safe because nutritional medicines, not pharmaceuticals, are employed. They are water-based highly concentrated nutritional medicines, not chemical, and the supreme ones are magnesium chloride, magnesium bicarbonate, sodium bicarbonate (baking soda), selenium, sulfur, iodine, and glutathione.

Vitamin C can be added to that list, but you unfortunately have to force doctors and hospitals, with legal process, to administer it intravenously when high dosages are needed. Court orders are effective in such cases and have been known to save lives because vitamin C is that useful in a medical pinch.

Every one of the above medicines can be used to great advantage not only for emergency situations but also for cancer, diabetes, the flu, neurological disorders, heart disease, and stroke. Few doctors or patients know how these medicinals can be used at home safely to treat ourselves and our loved ones. When used in combination with each other, they constitute a new form of medicine that is powerful yet easy to learn.

Anyone who sees and comprehends the potential medical horsepower of the full protocol will indeed realize what a powerful approach we have for giving everyone the best shot at not having to die from cancer. There are many ways to treat cancer, and combining the strongest and most necessary medicinals yields the best and most rational approach.

Anti-Inflammatory Oxygen Therapy

At the top of the protocol is the Tiger Tank of the medical world, which thrusts the entire protocol beyond anything seen or available in the world of medicine, health, anti-aging, sports, and beauty. The world of alkalinity and pH changed with the discovery that the *most important factor in creating proper pH is increasing oxygen.*

In my book *Anti-Inflammatory Oxygen Therapy* I introduce a new way of injecting massive amounts of oxygen into the cells, which will profoundly affect them. In fifteen minutes, one can blow the cells doors down allowing them to detoxify as they gulp down high levels of oxygen. The break-through is that it actually raises the arterial pressure back to youthful levels.

I have discovered a technique that offers much higher therapeutic results than an expensive, inconvenient hyperbaric chamber and can be done in your bedroom. A person needs an oxygen concentrator, exercise bicycle or rebounder, and a new mask kit with a reservoir that stores up enough O_2, before you even begin to use it, to supply the correct amount of oxygen needed for one fifteen minute session. It offers a trip to cellular heaven. This therapy is like putting out a candle flame with your fingers. In the first 15 minute session (or let's say first four sessions), the inflammation in the capillaries will be snubbed out and their toxins will be cleared. Oxygen will rush into the cells bringing the energy and the physiological processes necessary to heal.

Oxygen is all around us, but hardly anyone gets enough. It is a paradox that few understand, but it is the reason that sodium bicarbonate is such a wonderful medicine. It gives one instant access to more oxygen because the bicarbonates/CO_2 dilate the blood vessels, ensuring more blood and oxygen get delivered.

Below is an updated version of my protocol components. For the first time I bring onto one page not only an outline of the protocol, but links to the companies that sell the medicinals and medical devices.

1. Anti-Inflammatory Oxygen Therapy—LivO₂
LivO₂:
Website: http://liveO₂.com/
Call: Tom Butler at 970-658-2111
Email: tom@whnlive.com
Mailing address: Mark Squibb
                   PO Box 158
                   Bellvue, CO 80512

2. Bicarbonate/ Carbon Dioxide Medicine (sodium and potassium bicarbonates)

Bicarbonate Formula:

Forrest Health: call: 408-354-4262

Website: www.forresthealth.com

3. Magnesium Medicine:

Ancient Minerals Magnesium Oil:

LL's Magnetic Clay Co.

Contact in US: 800-257-3315

Customer service inquiries email: info@llmagneticclay.com

Website: www.ancient-minerals.com

Magnesium Bicarbonate Water:

Website: http://magbicarb.com

Contact: Cell: 407-963-8881 Skype: jaime.giroux

4. Iodine (with possible inclusion of natural thyroid hormone)

Nascent Iodine:

LL's Magnetic Clay Co.

Contact in USA: 1-800-257-3315

Customer service inquiries email: info@llmagneticclay.com

Website: www.magneticclay.com

5. Liquid Selenium

Call: Tom Butler at 970-658-2111

Email: tom@whnlive.com

Mailing address: Mark Squibb

PO Box 158

Bellvue, CO 80512

Website: http://care.whnlive.com

6. Vitamin E

UNIQUE Optimum E Complex:

Website: www.amazon.com

7. Glutathione

Sublingual; ACG Glutathione Extra Strength Spray:

Forrest Health: call: 408-354-4262

Website: www.forresthealth.com

Nebulization: Reduced L-Glutathione Plus:
Theranaturals, Inc
P.O. Box 762
Nampa, ID 83653
Phone (Toll-Free): 866-435-659
(Direct): 435-671-4205
Email: theranat@fiber.net
Website: www.theranaturals.com

Suppositories: Glutathione (Reduced) Suppositories:
Forrest Health: call: 408-354-4262
Website: www.forresthealth.com

8. Cannabidiol (CBD) (legalized medical marijuana without THC) (THC where it is legal)
Dixie Botanicals
4990 Oakland St.
Denver, Co 80239
Phone: Toll-Free: 866-920-4262
Website: http://dixiebotanicals.com

9. Far-Infrared BioMats (treatments for cancer and pain) via Medical BioMats
Contact via on-line form: www.medicalbiomats.com
Website: www.medicalbiomats.com

10. Breathing retraining (slowing the breathing down, cancer treatment, stress reduction)
Blowing Bubbles—Revolutionary Cancer Treatment: by Dr. Mark Sircus
http://drsircus.com

Breathe Slim, Inc.
Buffalo Grove, IL 60089, U.S.A.
Customer Service (Call Toll Free): 866-Slim Slim (754-6754)
For local and international calls: +1-847-850-5800
Website: www.breathslim.com

11. *Tears of the Melting Heart* (connecting directly with one's own vulnerability)
By Dr. Mark Sircus

Website: http://drsircus.com

12. Vitamin C (high ORAC antioxidant therapy)
Ultimate Protector
Health Products Distributors, Inc.
Call toll-free: 800-228-4265
Local Arizona: 520-896-9193
Email: support@integratedhealth.com

13. Sun exposure, vitamin D
Vitamin D3 Plus:
Health Products Distributors, Inc.
Call toll-free: 800-228-4265
Local Arizona: 520-896-9193
Email: support@integratedhealth.com
Website: www.integratedhealth.com

14. Bioresonance Therapy (frequency medicine from Deta ESlis)
Deta Elis—*Star Trek Medicine—Bioresonance,* by Dr. Mark Sircus:
Website: http://drsircus.com
Deta Elis:
Website: www.deta-elis-uk.com
Email: admin@deta-elis-uk.com
Contact: via online form: www.deta-elis-uk.com

15. Water (medicinal quality and full hydration)

16. Sexual Healing and Health
Love & Sex Medicine ebook by Dr. Mark Sircus
Website: http://drsircus.com

17. Nutrition
Super foods:
Rejuvenate
Website: www.integratedhealth.com
Call: 800-228-4265
Local Arizona: 520-896-9193
Email: support@integratedhealth.com

Hydrochloric acid:
Betaine Hydrochloride

Website: http://care.whnlive.com
Call: Tom Butler at 970-658-2111
Email: tom@whnlive.com
Mailing address: Mark Squibb
                      PO Box 158
                      Bellvue, CO 80512

Natural Chelation:
Heavy Metal Detox
Website: www.detoxmetals.com
Call: US/Worldwide: (+1)866-508-8357
Email: admin@detoxmetals.com

Enzyme therapy:
Prolyte
Health Products Distributors, Inc.
Toll-free: 800-228-4265
Local Arizona: 520-896-9193
Email: support@integratedhealth.com
Website: www.integratedhealth.com
Vitamins A & B, juice fasting:

Aloe vera—*Body Balance*
Website: http://lifeforce.net

Organic Sulfur (MSM):
Email: mail@organic-sulfur.com
Website: www.organic-sulfur.com

Alpha-lipoic acid, sodium thiosulfate, seawater

18. Intestinal health

Probiotics:
Prescript Assist
LL's Magnetic Clay Co.
Contact in USA: 1-800-257-3315
Customer service inquiries email: info@llmagneticclay.com
website: www.prescript-assist.com

Enemas, colonics:
Clay: Edible Earth
LL's Magnetic Clay Co.
Contact in USA: 1-800-257-3315

Customer service inquiries email: info@llmagneticclay.com
Website: www.magneticclay.com

19. Exercise, yoga
(Social support, therapeutic support, therapeutic massage, spiritual processing, abdominal shiatsu)

20. Ayahuasca, Mistletoe
Ayahuasca by Dr. Mark Sircus
Website: http://drsircus.com
Mistletoe (Viscum album)
Website: www.bmj.com

References

Introduction

1 *International Journal of Food Microbiology*. Volume 109, Issues 1–2, 25 May 2006, Pages 160–163. Virucidal efficacy of sodium bicarbonate on a food contact surface against feline calicivirus, a norovirus surrogate Yashpal S. Malik and Sagar M. Goyal. Department of Veterinary Population Medicine, College of Veterinary Medicine, University of Minnesota. The virucidal efficacy of sodium bicarbonate was enhanced when it was used in combination with aldehydes or hydrogen peroxide.

2 Sodium bicarbonate 50mmol in each Liter of IV hydration fluid and/or sodium bicarbonate 1000mg/m2 PO q6h. Post-Chemotherapy Treatments: Serum Methotrexate levels—30 minutes after infusion ends; q12h intervals from the start of the infusion x 2; then at 0800H daily for at least one day. For hydration: Continue IV fluid at 100–125mL/hour, to maintain urine output >60mL/hr. Measure strict in and out q1h x 24 hrs. For alkalinization: Continue pre-chemo alkalinization for 24 hours after infusion ends. www.cancercare.on.ca/pdfchemo/hdmtx-osteo.pdf

3 "Enhancement of chemotherapy by manipulation of tumourpH." Raghunand N, He X, van Sluis R, Mahoney B, Baggett B, Taylor CW, Paine-Murrieta G, Roe D, Bhujwalla ZM, Gillies RJ. Arizona Cancer Center.

4 www.cancerbackup.org.uk/Treatments/Chemotherapy/Combinationregimen/Hyper-CVAD

5 This drug is highly toxic and both powder and solution must be handled and administered with care. Inhalation of dust or vapors and contact with skin or mucous membranes, especially those of the eyes, must be avoided. Due to the toxic properties of mechlorethamine (e. g., corrosivity, carcinogenicity, mutagenicity, teratogenicity), special handling procedures should be reviewed prior to handling and followed diligently. Extravasation of the drug into subcutaneous tissues results in a painful inflammation. The area usually becomes indurated and sloughing may occur. If leakage of drug is obvious, prompt infiltration of the area with sterile isotonic sodium thiosulfate (1/6 molar) and application of an ice compress for 6 to 12 hours may minimize the local reaction. For a 1/6 molar solution of sodium thiosulfate, use 4.14 g of sodium thiosulfate per 100 mL of Sterile Water for Injection or 2.64 g of anhydrous sodium thiosulfate per 100 mL or dilute 4 mL of Sodium Thiosulfate Injection (10percent) with 6 mL of Sterile Water for Injection.

Chapter 1

1 *International Journal of Food Microbiology.* Volume 109, Issues 1–2, 25 May 2006, Pages 160–163. Virucidal efficacy of sodium bicarbonate on a food contact surface against feline calicivirus, a norovirus surrogate Yashpal S. Malik and Sagar M. Goyal. Department of Veterinary Population Medicine, College of Veterinary Medicine, University of Minnesota. The virucidal efficacy of sodium bicarbonate was enhanced when it was used in combination with aldehydes or hydrogen peroxide.

2 Enzymes are protein catalysts that influence the rate of a reaction. The reactant substances upon which an enzyme acts are termed the substrates. The substances produced as a result of the reaction are the products. Enzyme-controlled reactions are mostly reversible and involve the formation of an intermediate enzyme-substrate complex.

3 "Acute inflammation alters bicarbonate transport in mouse ileum." *The Journal of Physiology.* March 1, 2010, 588 (5) Hui Zhang, Nadia Ameen, James E. Melvin and Sadasivan-Vidyasagar

4 Okamura *et al.* 1985, Speroffet al. 1994.

5 http://sciencelinks.jp/j-east/article/200421/000020042104A0734385.php

Chapter 2

1"Bicarbonate Transport in Cell Physiology and Disease." Emmanuelle Cordat and Joseph R. Casey. Membrane Protein Research Group, Department of Physiology1 and Department of Biochemistry2 University of Alberta, Edmonton Canada T6G 2H7

2 Gas bubbles in carbonated water are created by adding carbon dioxide to plain water. Carbonated water does not contain phosphoric acid, which strips bones of calcium and causes blood acidity. Carbonated water has one ingredient that soft drinks lack: bicarbonate. Bicarbonate minimizes calcium loss from the bones. Since blood acidity is not excessive when consuming carbonated water due to bicarbonate, more calcium stays in the bones.

3 *American Society for Nutritional Sciences J.Nutr.*134:1058–1063, May 2004

4 *Journal of Sports Science and Medicine,* March 1, 2009. Zajac, Adam; Cholewa, Jaroslaw; Poprzecki, Stanislaw; Waskiewicz, Zbigniew; Langfort, Jozef

Chapter 3

1 A complex structure adhering to surfaces that are regularly in contact with water, consisting of colonies of bacteria and other microorganisms such as yeasts, fungi, and protozoa that secrete a mucilaginous protective coating in which they are encased. Biofilms can form on solid or liquid surfaces as well as on soft tissue in living organisms, and are typically resistant to conventional methods of disinfection. Dental plaque, the slimy coating that fouls pipes and tanks, and algal mats on bodies of water are examples of biofilms.

2 Sodium bicarbonate 5 percent ear drops. Age from 6 months onwards. Sodium bicarbonate ear drops. Put 3 to 4 drops into the affected ear(s) 3 to 4 times a day for 3 to 5 days. http://cks.library.nhs.uk/earwax/view_whole_guidance Alternate and use with iodine to combat ear infections.

3 Buysse CMP, de Jongste JC, de Hoog M. "Life-threatening asthma in children: treat-

ment with sodium bicarbonate reduces PCO_2. Chest." 2005;127:866–870. www.pulmonaryreviews.com/jun05/sodium.html

Corinne M. P. Buysse, MD, and colleagues retrospectively evaluated the use of sodium bicarbonate in 17 children with life-threatening asthma. Sixteen of these children had acidosis, indicating severe respiratory distress. The acidosis was classified as mixed respiratory and metabolic in 13 patients, predominantly respiratory in one patient, and metabolic in two patients. In one patient, the initial blood gas values before administration of sodium bicarbonate in the referring hospital could not be traced. A new protocol was initiated using IV magnesium sulfate and IV sodium bicarbonate as adjunctive therapy when respiratory distress persisted despite standard treatment. According to Dr. Buysse, a pediatric intensivist at the Erasmus MC–Sophia Children's Hospital in Rotterdam, Netherlands, "Administration of sodium bicarbonate was associated with a significant decrease in PCO_2 in 17 children with life-threatening asthma. Improvement of respiratory distress was observed as well."

4 www.pccmjournal.com/pt/re/pccm/abstract.00130478–200703000–00016.htm;jsessionid=LftNGWdNXk8fRr0qDpdfkhgrCQv9J5NGSPxffZnGHNpJ5mTY7sXQ!542054210!181195628!8091!-1

5 http://clinicaltrials.gov/show/NCT01426165

6 *Health Affairs*, 29, no. 2 (2010): 324–326 doi: 10.1377/hlthaff.2009.0407

7 These include, Benzotropines (valium) cyclic antidepressants (amytriptayine), organophosphates, methanol (Methyl alcohol is a cheap and potent adulterant of illicit liquors) Diphenhydramine (Benedryl), Beta blockers (propanalol) Barbiturates, and Salicylates (Aspirin). Poisoning by drugs that block voltage-gated sodium channels produces intraventricular conduction defects, myocardial depression, bradycardia, and ventricular arrhythmias. Human and animal reports suggest that hypertonic sodium bicarbonate may be effective therapy for numerous agents possessing sodium channel blocking properties, including cocaine, quinidine, procainamide, flecainide, mexiletine, bupivacaine, and others.

8 Gamba, G., "Bicarbonate therapy in severe diabetic ketoacidosis. A double blind, randomized, placebo controlled trial." (*Rev Invest Clin* 1991 Jul-Sep;43(3):234–8). Miyares Gomez A. in "Diabetic ketoacidosis in childhood: the first day of treatment (*An EspPediatr* 1989 Apr;30(4):279–83)

9 Levy, M.M., "An evidence-based evaluation of the use of sodium bicarbonate during cardiopulmonary resuscitation" (Crit Care Clin 1998 Jul;14(3):457–83). Vukmir, R.B., Sodium bicarbonate in cardiac arrest: a reappraisal (*Am J Emerg Med* 1996 Mar;14(2):192–206). Bar-Joseph, G., "Clinical use of sodium bicarbonate during cardiopulmonary resuscitation—is it used sensibly?" (Resuscitation 2002 Jul;54(1):47–55).

10 Zhang. L.,"Perhydrit and sodium bicarbonate improve maternal gases and acid-base status during the second stage of labor" Department of Obstetrics and Gynecology, Xiangya Hospital, Hunan Medical University, Changsha 410008. Maeda, Y., "Perioperative administration of bicarbonated solution to a patient with mitochondrial encephalomyopathy" (*Masui* 2001 Mar;50(3):299–303).

11 Avdic. E., "Bicarbonate versus acetate hemodialysis: effects on the acid-base status" (*Med Arh* 2001;55(4):231–3).

12 Feriani, M., "Randomized long-term evaluation of bicarbonate-buffered CAPD solution." (*Kidney Int* 1998 Nov;54(5):1731–8).

13 Vrijlandt, P.J., "Sodium bicarbonate infusion for intoxication with tricyclic antidepressives: recommended inspite of lack of scientific evidence" *Ned TijdschrGeneeskd* 2001 Sep 1;145(35):1686–9). Knudsen, K., "Epinephrine and sodium bicarbonate independently and additively increase survival in experimental amitriptyline poisoning." (*Crit Care Med* 1997 Apr;25(4):669–74).

14 Silomon, M., "Effect of sodium bicarbonate infusion on hepatocyte Ca2+ overload during resuscitation from hemorrhagic shock." (Resuscitation 1998 Apr;37(1):27–32). Mariano, F., "Insufficient correction of blood bicarbonate levels in biguanide lactic acidosis treated with CVVH and bicarbonate replacement fluids" (*Minerva UrolNefrol* 1997 Sep;49(3):133–6).

15 Dement'eva, I.I., "Calculation of the dose of sodium bicarbonate in the treatment of metabolic acidosis in surgery with and deep hypothermic circulatory arrest" (*AnesteziolReanimatol* 1997 Sep-Oct;(5):42–4).

Chapter 4

[1] "Origin of the Bicarbonate Stimulation of Torpedo Electric Organ Synaptic Vesicle ATPase." Joan E. Rothlein 1 Stanley M. Parsons. Department of Chemistry and the Marine Science Institute, University of California, Santa Barbara, Santa Barbara, California, U.S.A.

[2] www.docstoc.com/docs/24767241/Allergy-Effects-On-The-Pancreas-And-Small-Intestine/

[3] Epithelial cells in pancreatic ducts are the source of the bicarbonate and water secreted by the pancreas. Bicarbonate is a base and critical to neutralizing the acid coming into the small intestine from the stomach. The mechanism underlying bicarbonate secretion is essentially the same as for acid secretion parietal cells and is dependent on the enzyme carbonic anhydrase. In pancreatic duct cells, the bicarbonate is secreted into the lumen of the duct and hence into pancreatic juice.

[4] *Brain Allergies: The Psychonutrient and Magnetic Connections.* By William Philpott, Dwight K. Kalita Published by McGraw-Hill Professional, 2000

[5] "Impaired pancreatic bicarbonate secretion in chronic malnutrition." *Indian pediatrics* ISSN 0019–6061 1995, vol. 32, no3, pp. 323–329 (24 ref.)

[6]www.remm.nlm.gov/int_contamination.htm

Chapter 5

[1] "A study of the acidosis, blood urea, and plasma chlorides in uranium nephritis in the dog, and the protective action of sodium bicarbonate." *The Journal of Experimental Medicine,* Vol 25, 693–719, Copyright, 1917, by The Rockefeller Institute for Medical Research New York www.jem.org/cgi/content/abstract/25/5/693

[2] Levine DZ, Jacobson HR: "The regulation of renal acid secretion: New observations from studies of distal nephron segments." *Kidney Int*29:1099–1109, 1986

[3]JAMA 2004;291:2328–2334,2376–2377.

www.urotoday.com/56/browse_categories/renal_transplantation_vascular_disease/so
dium_bicarbonate_may_prevent_radiocontrastinduced_renal_injury.html

4 www.uptodate.com/patients/content/abstract.do?topicKey=~G/p55S8w8sQD-
wqG&refNum=28

5 www.ncbi.nlm.nih.gov/pubmed/16523427

6 http://news.bbc.co.uk/2/hi/health/7655405.stm

7 These include, Benzotropines (valium) cyclic antidepressants (amytriptayine),
organophosphates, methanol (Methyl alcohol is a cheap and potent adulterant of illicit
liquors) Diphenhydramine (Benedryl), Beta blockers (propanalol) Barbiturates, and Salicylates (Aspirin). Poisoning by drugs that block voltage-gated sodium channels produces intraventricular conduction defects, myocardial depression, bradycardia, and
ventricular arrhythmias. Human and animal reports suggest that hypertonic sodium
bicarbonate may be effective therapy for numerous agents possessing sodium channel
blocking properties, including cocaine, quinidine, procainamide, flecainide, mexiletine,
bupivacaine, and others.

8 *Perit Dial Int* 11(3): 224–227 *Peritoneal Dialysis International*, Vol 11, Issue 3, 224–227

9 *Am J ClinNutr* 1998;68:576–83.

Estimation of net endogenous noncarbonic acid production in humans from diet potassium and protein contents1–3.

Lynda A Frassetto, Karen M Todd, R Curtis Morris Jr, and Anthony Sebastian

10 Frassetto L, Sebastian A. "Age and systemic acid-base equilibrium: analysis of published data." J Gerontol 1996:51A:B91–9.

11 Lindeman RD, Tobin J, Shock NW. "Longitudinal studies on the rate of decline in
renal function with age." *J AmGeriatrSoc* 1985; 33:278–85.

12 Torres VE, Cowley BD, Branden MG, Yoshida I, Gattone VH. Nephrology Research
Unit and Division of Nephrology, Mayo Clinic, Rochester, Minn 55905, USA. *ExpNephrol.*
2001;9(3):171–80. torres.vicente@mayo.edu.

Chapter 6

1 Old fashioned sodium bicarbonate baths for the treatment of psoriasis in the era of
futuristic biologics: An old ally to be rescued; *Journal of Dermatological Treatment;* Volume
16, Number 1/February 2005.

2 http://cgi.ebay.com/ARM-&-HAMMER-BAKING-SODA-MEDICAL-USES-
BROCHURE-1924_W0QQitemZ370285074486QQcmdZViewItemQQimsxZ20091104?
IMSfp=TL091104191005r1063

3 A testimonial left on my site by Laurel from Australia.

4 Secretion of bicarbonate into the adherent layer of mucus gel creates a pH gradient
with a near-neutral pH at the epithelial surfaces in stomach and duodenum, providing
the first line of mucosal protection against luminal acid. The continuous adherent mucus
layer is also a barrier to luminal pepsin, thereby protecting the underlying mucosa from
proteolytic digestion.

5 www.mgwater.com/bicarb.shtml.

6 The pH of the stomach may go as low as 1.0. This is a very acidic level. Because the pH

scale is a logarithmic scale, the pH of the stomach is hundreds or thousands or millions of times stronger than typical cellular fluids which are generally close to 7.0 (the neutral level on the pH scale.) When food comes into the stomach, the pH may rise to levels in the 3.0 to 4.0 level due to the buffering capacity of proteins. Solutions at a pH of 1.0 are strong enough to burn through fabrics, injure eyes or irritate skin.

[7] *News* vol 3, no 1, May 2001.

[8] http://en.wikipedia.org/wiki/William–Beaumont.

[9] A complex structure adhering to surfaces that are regularly in contact with water, consisting of colonies of bacteria and other microorganisms such as yeasts, fungi, and protozoa that secrete a mucilaginous protective coating in which they are encased. Biofilms can form on solid or liquid surfaces as well as on soft tissue in living organisms, and are typically resistant to conventional methods of disinfection. Dental plaque, the slimy coating that fouls pipes and tanks, and algal mats on bodies of water are examples of biofilms.

[10] "A Prospective Study of Periodontal Disease and Pancreatic Cancer in U.S. Male Health Professionals." Dominique S. Michaud, KaumudiJoshipura, Edward Giovannucci, and Charles S. Fuchs. *J. Natl. Cancer Inst.* 2007 99: 171–175; doi:10.1093/jnci/djk021

[11] www.healingdaily.com/conditions/bleeding-gums.htm

[12] Tezal M, Sullivan M, Reid M, et al. "Chronic Periodontitis and the risk of tongue cancer." *Archives of Otolaryngology – Head and Neck Surgery.* 2007; 133:450–454

[13] www.ncl.ac.uk/dental/research/oral/periodontal.htm

[14] www.cancer.gov/cancertopics/pdq/supportivecare/oralcomplications/HealthProfessional/page5/print

Chapter 7

[1] *Cancer Research* 69, 2677, March 15, 2009. Published Online First March 10, 2009; doi: 10.1158/0008–5472.CAN-08–2394

[2] www.ncbi.nlm.nih.gov/pubmed/19276390

[3] The breakdown of glucose or glycogen produces lactate and hydrogen ions—for each lactate molecule, one hydrogen ion is formed. The presence of hydrogen ions, not lactate, makes the muscle acidic that will eventually halt muscle function. As hydrogen ion concentrations increase the blood and muscle become acidic. This acidic environment will slow down enzyme activity and ultimately the breakdown of glucose itself. Acidic muscles will aggravate associated nerve endings causing pain and increase irritation of the central nervous system. The athlete may become disorientated and feel nauseous.

[4] By buffering acidity in the blood, bicarbonate draws more of the acid produced within the muscle cells out into the blood and thus reduce the level of acidity within the muscle cells themselves.

Chapter 8

[1] Mazzotti, E. et al. "Treatment-related side effects and quality of life in cancer patients." *Supportive Care in Cancer.* 2011. doi: 10.1007/s00520–011–1354-y. Online first.

2 www.dailymail.co.uk/health/article-2100684/Why-doctors-like-die-endure-pain-treatment-advanced-cancer.html

3 *Gofman, John; Preventing Breast Cancer;* San Francisco; The Comittee for Nuclear Responsibility;1995

4 "A study of the acidosis, blood urea, and plasma chlorides in uranium nephritis in the dog, and the protective action of sodium bicarbonate." *The Journal of Experimental Medicine,* Vol 25, 693–719, Copyright, 1917, by The Rockefeller Institute for Medical Research New York www.jem.org/cgi/content/abstract/25/5/693

5 Ibid

Chapter 9

1 Henderson, Y. "Carbon Dioxide." Article in Encyclopedia of Medicine. 1940.

2 By Dr. Gerald Marsh:Five hundred million years ago, carbon dioxide concentrations were over 13 times current levels; and not until about 20 million years ago did carbon dioxide levels dropped to a little less than twice what they are today. It is possible that moderately increased carbon dioxide concentrations could extend the current interglacial period. But we have not reached the level required yet, nor do we know the optimum level to reach. So, rather than call for arbitrary limits on carbon dioxide emissions, perhaps the best thing the UN's Intergovernmental Panel on Climate Change and the climatology community in general could do is spend their efforts on determining the optimal range of carbon dioxide needed to extend the current interglacial period indefinitely. We ought to carefully consider this possibility before we wipe out our current prosperity by spending trillions of dollars to combat a perceived global warming threat that may well prove to be only a will-o-the-wisp.Dr. Gerald Marsh is a retired physicist from the Argonne National Laboratory and a former consultant to the Department of Defense on strategic nuclear technology and policy in the Reagan, Bush, and Clinton Administration.

3www.medicalnewstoday.com/articles/159225.php

4 *BMJ.* 1998 November 7; 317(7168): 1302–1306

5 J. Cui, X. Mao, V. Olman, P. J. Hastings, Y. Xu. "Hypoxia and miscoupling between reduced energy efficiency and signaling to cell proliferation drive cancer to grow increasingly faster." *Journal of Molecular Cell Biology,* 2012; DOI:10.1093/jmcb/mjs017

6 M. Milosevic, P. Warde, C. Menard, P. Chung, A. Toi, A. Ishkanian, M. McLean, M. Pintilie, J. Sykes, M. Gospodarowicz, C. Catton, R. P. Hill, R. Bristow. "Tumor Hypoxia Predicts Biochemical Failure following Radiotherapy for Clinically Localized Prostate Cancer." *Clinical Cancer Research,* 2012; 18 (7): 2108 DOI:10.1158/1078–0432.CCR-11–2711

7 Rockwell S, "Oxygen delivery: implications for the biology and therapy of solid tumors," *Oncology Research* 1997; 9(6–7): p. 383–390.

8 "Temporal, spatial, and oxygen-regulated expression of hypoxia-inducible factor-1 in the lung;" Aimee Y.Yu1et al; *AJP - Lung Physiol;* October 1, 1998 vol. 275 no. 4 L818-L826

9 Shaw, K. (2008) "Environmental cues like hypoxia can trigger gene expression and cancer development." *Nature Education* 1(1)

10 The Regulation of HIF-1http://molpharm.aspetjournals.org/content/70/5/1469.full#sec-3

11 Grocery Store Baking Soda; A Source of Sodium Bicarbonate in the Management of Chronic Metabolic Acidosis; Oral sodium bicarbonate is used to treat metabolic acidosis in patients with renal tubular acidosis. Since infants and young children are unable to swallow tablets, those affected must ingest sodium bicarbonate in a powder or liquid form. Pharmacy-weighed sodium bicarbonate is expensive and inconvenient to obtain; some pharmacists are reluctant to provide it. We determined that the sodium bicarbonate contained in 8-oz boxes of Arm & Hammer Baking Soda® was sufficiently constant in weight that, dissolved in water to a given volume, it yielded a quantitatively acceptable therapeutic solution of sodium bicarbonate at a cost of approximately 3 percent of that of pharmacy-weighed sodium bicarbonate.http://cpj.sagepub.com/content/23/2/94.abstract

12 *Cancer Research 69, 2677,* March 15, 2009. Published Online First March 10, 2009;doi: 10.1158/0008–5472.CAN-08–2394

13 *Cancer Research* 2009;69(6):2260–8

14 *www.ncbi.nlm.nih.gov/entrez/query.fcgi?cmd=Retrieve&db=PubMed&list_uids= 10362108&dopt=Abstract*

Chapter 10

1 Henderson, Y. "Carbon Dioxide." Article in Encyclopedia of Medicine. 1940.

2 http://raypeat.com/articles/aging/altitude-mortality.shtml

3 www.positivehealth.com/article-view.php?articleid=1436

4 "Chloride-Bicarbonate Exchange in Red Blood Cells: Physiology of Transport and Chemical Modification of Binding Site." Wieth, J. O.; Andersen, O. S.; Brahm, J.; Bjerrum, P. J.; Borders, C. L., Jr. Philosophical Transactions of the Royal Society of London. Series B, *Biological Sciences,* Volume 299, Issue 1097, pp. 383–399

5 www.fishchannel.com/saltwater-aquariums/aquarium-frontiers/CO_2-friend-or-foe.aspx?cm_sp=InternalClicks-_-RelatedArticles-_-saltwater-aquariums/aquarium-frontiers/CO_2-friend-or-foe

6 "Stimulation by sparkling water of gastroduodenal HCO_3^- secretion in rats." *Medical Science Monitor.* 2009 Dec;15(12):BR349–56. Division of Pathological Sciences, Department of Pharmacology and Experimental Therapeutics, Kyoto Pharmaceutical University, Misasagi, Yamashina, Kyoto, Japan.

Chapter 11

1 "Enhancement of chemotherapy by manipulation of tumourpH."Raghunand N, He X, van Sluis R, Mahoney B, Baggett B, Taylor CW, Paine-Murrieta G, Roe D, Bhujwalla ZM, Gillies RJ. Arizona Cancer Center, Tucson 85724–5024, USA.

2 www.urotoday.com/38/browse_categories/renal_cancer/sodium_bicarbonate_infusion_found_to_reduce_risk_of_contrastinduced_nephropathy.html

3 http://news.bbc.co.uk/2/hi/health/7655405.stm

4 Jerome B. Westin and Elihu Richter, "The Israeli Breast-Cancer Anomaly," in Devra Lee Davis and David Hoel, editors, "Trends in Cancer Mortality in Industrial Countries" (New York: New York Academy of Sciences, 1990), pgs. 269–279. Following public outcry, Israel banned these chemicals from being used on feed for dairy cows and cattle.

Over the next ten years, the rate of breast cancer deaths in Israel declined sharply, with a 30 percent drop in mortality for women under 44 years of age, and an 8percent overall decline. At the same time, all other known cancer risks—alcohol consumption, fat intake, lack of fruits and vegetables in the diet—increased significantly. During this period, worldwide death rates from cancer increased by 4percent. The only answer scientists could find to explain this was the reduced level of environmental toxins.

5 "A mass spectrographic analysis of cancer cells showed that the cell membrane readily attached cesium, rubidium and potassium, and transmitted these elements with their associated molecules into the cancer cell. In contrast cancer membranes did not transmit sodium, magnesium, and calcium into the cell: the amount of calcium within a cancer cell is only about 1percent of that for normal cells. Potassium transports glucose into the cell. Calcium and magnesium transport oxygen into the cell. As a consequence of the above, oxygen cannot enter cancer cells so the glucose which is normally burned to carbon dioxide and water undergoes fermentation to form lactic acid within the cell. This anaerobic condition was pointed out by Warburg, as early as 1924. Potassium, and especially rubidium and cesium are the most basic of the elements. When they are taken up by the cancer cells they will thus raise the pH of the cells. Since they are very strong bases as compared to the weak lactic acid it is possible that the pH will be raised to values in the 8.5 to 9 range. In this range the life of the cancer cell is short, being a matter of days at the most. The dead cancer cells are then absorbed by the body fluids and eventually eliminated from the system." - Dr. Brewerwww.mwt.net/~drbrewer/highpH.htm

6 Lee, H., Cha, M., Kim, I. "Activation of thiol-dependant antioxidant activity of human serum albumin by alkaline pH is due to the b-like conformational change."

Chapter 12

1 There has been considerable interest in the use of baking soda (sodium bicarbonate, $NaHCO_3$) and potassium bicarbonate ($KHCO_3$) to control powdery mildew and other fungal diseases of plants. The use of baking soda as a fungicide is not a new idea. In Alfred C. Hottes' *A Little Book of Climbing Plants*, published in 1933 by the A.T. De La Mare Co. of New York, mention is made of using one ounce of baking soda per gallon of water to control powdery mildew (PM) on climbing roses. The author credits the idea to a Russian plant pathologist, A. de Yaczenski. In the August, 1985 issue of *Organic Gardening* magazine, a short article by Warren Shultz entitled "Recipe for Resistance" reports that researchers in Japan obtained effective control of PM on cucumbers, eggplants, and strawberries. They suggested weekly sprays of $1/4$ ounce baking soda per gallon of water. An article in the June, 1990 issue of *Greenhouse Manager* magazine summarizes the results of three years of testing baking soda as a fungicide for roses. Cornell University researcher Dr. R. Kenneth Horst observed suppression of PM and blackspot—both major problems for New York rose growers. Roses were sprayed every 3 to 4 days with a water solution of baking soda and insecticidal soap.

http://attra.ncat.org/attra-pub/bakingsoda.html

2 "Sodium Carbonate and Sodium bicarbonate were equal and superior to the other salts for control of green mold on oranges." *CommunAgricApplBiol Sci.* 2007;72(4):773–7.

3 "Chronic Fatigue Immune Dysfunction Syndrome (CFIDS)" Also Referred to as:"Yeast Syndrome or Yeast Related Illness" by Elmer M. Cranton, M.D.; Copyright © 2007 Elmer M. Cranton, M.D.

4 Jack D. Sobel, MD. "Candidal Vulvovaginitis," *Clinical Obstetrics and Gynecology*, 1993 Vol.36 (1): 153–165

5 Velicer C, et al. *JAMA*. Feb 2004. 18;291(7):827–35

6 *Medical Tribune:* "Treatment of Fungal Infections Led to Leukemia Remission." Sept 29, 1999; Mann, D. Antifungal agent lowers PSA levels, study finds. May 1, 1997.

7 Moore-Landecker, *Fundamentals of Fungi*, 4th ed. 1996; AND Shim, H. , et al. A unique glucose-dependent apoptotic pathway induced by c-Myc. Proceedings of the National Academy of Science. 95;1511–1516. 1998

8 Ochmanski, W., et al. PrzeglLek 2000;57(7–8):419–23

9 www.cancerfightingstrategies.com/fungalconnection.html

10 The National Academies Press. "Toxicological Effects of Methylmercury" (2000) Commission on Life Sciences

11 "The Pathogenic Multi-potency of Mercury, Biological Therapy," *Journal of Natural Medicine*, Vol. VI, No. 3, June 1988

12 www.abc.net.au/news/stories/2006/06/15/1663938.htm

13 Takeuchi H, Arai Y, Konami T, Ikeda T, Tomoyoshi T, Tatewaki K. Hinyokika Kiyo. 1983 Oct;29(10):1273–7.

14 www.vaccinetruth.org/is_cancer_contagious.htm

15 The regulatory limits of aflatoxin are 0.5 ppb and 20 ppb for milk and grain products intended for food consumption, but livestock feed is allowed to contain aflatoxin up to 300 ppb, which greatly increases the amounts of aflotoxins in our diets. Dietary restrictions are inadequate to protect us andmycotoxins are even on the skins of some fruits and in some areas of world, are problematic in drinking water.

16 Kemin.com; Kemin Americas Inc; "The Control of Mold and Mycotoxins In Ruminant Feeds;" Dec. 2002.

17 Council for Agricultural Science and Technology. Mycotoxins: "Risks in Plant, Animal and Human Systems Task Force Report;" number 139.CAST Ames, IA; Jan.2003

18 *Infectious Diabetes;* Kaufman and Holland; Chapter 3: The Fungus Among Us.

19 Enlargement of a part due to an abnormal numerical increase of its cells.

20 Dr. David Holland wrote that in 1999 Dr. MeinolfKarthaus watched three different children with leukemia suddenly go into remission upon receiving a triple antifungal drug cocktail for their "secondary" fungal infections. Pre-dating that, Mark Bielski stated back in 1997 that leukemia, whether acute or chronic, is intimately associated with the yeast, Candida albicans. Dr. J. Walter Wilson, in his textbook of clinical mycology a half a century ago said that "it has been established that histoplasmosis and such reticuloendothelioses as leukemia, Hodgkin's disease, lymphosarcoma, and sarcoidosis are found to be coexistent much more frequently than is statistically justifiable on the basis of coincidence." Histoplasmosis is what we call an "endemic" fungal infection. The late Dr. Milton White believed that cancer is a "chronic, intracellular, infectious, biologically induced spore (fungus) transformation disease."

21 www.cancer.med.umich.edu/news/stemcell.shtml

22 www.dundee.ac.uk/pressoffice/contact/2007/june/fungi.html

23 To ascertain the importance of fungi ingestion on heavy metal intake in roe deer, we simultaneously studied fungal spores (by microscopic determination) and heavy metal levels (by inductively coupled plasma mass spectrometry and atomic absorption spectrometry) in roe deer faeces, collected in the period July-November 2001 at VelikiVrh, the Salek Valley, Slovenia. Irrespective of species, fungal spores were present in 89percent of faeces; the following genera were found to be consumed by roe deer: Lycoperdon, Calvatia, Hypholoma, Coprinus, Russula, Elaphomyces, Xeromomus, Enteloma, Amanita, Cortinarius, Agaricus, Inocybe, Boletus, Macrolepiota, Suillus and Pluteus. While the importance of fungi ingestion on the seasonal variability of other metals is less clear, it doubtless influences Hg intake in roe deer, which is confirmed by: (a) the high frequency of fungi in roe deer nutrition; (b) their hyperaccumulative ability; (c) the temporal distribution of Hg in roe deer faeces; (d) differences among three classes of faeces established on the basis of the frequency of spores present; (e) the correlation between the number of fungal genera present and Hg levels in faeces. Therefore, the influence of fungi ingestion has to be taken into consideration in assessing the hazard due to the accumulation of mercury along the food-chain. Fungi ingestion as an important factor influencing heavy metal intake in roe deer: evidence from faeces; Pokorny, B et al; *Sci Total Environ.* 2004 May 25;324(1–3):223–34

24 www.osti.gov/energycitations/product.biblio.jsp?osti_id=5661650

Chapter 13

1 Side effects wear off quickly but can include racing pulse, tremors, nausea and insomnia. Nebulizer asthma treatments can also raise blood pressure and aggravate glaucoma.

2 http://kidshealth.org/parent/medical/asthma/inhaler_nebulizer.html

3 www.emedmag.com/html/pre/tox/0804.asp

Chapter 14

1 www.pccmjournal.com/pt/re/pccm/abstract.00130478–200703000–00016.htm;jsessionid=LftNGWdNXk8fRr0qDpdfkhgrCQv9J5NGSPxffZnGHNpJ5mTY7sXQ!54205421 0!181195628!8091!-1

2These include, Benzotropines (valium) cyclic antidepressants (amytriptayine), organophosphates, methanol (Methyl alcohol is a cheap and potent adulterant of illicit liquors) Diphenhydramine (Benedryl), Beta blockers (propanalol) Barbiturates, and Salicylates (Aspirin). Poisoning by drugs that block voltage-gated sodium channels produces intraventricular conduction defects, myocardial depression, bradycardia, and ventricular arrhythmias. Human and animal reports suggest that hypertonic sodium bicarbonate may be effective therapy for numerous agents possessing sodium channel blocking properties, including cocaine, quinidine, procainamide, flecainide, mexiletine, bupivacaine, and others.

3 www.mgwater.com/bicarb.shtml

Chapter 15

1 www.earthclinic.com/Remedies/molasses.html

2 The average of the five days of saliva pH will give you an idea whether your physiology is being dominated by emotions. If emotional overload is a factor, this also needs

to be addressed to prevent the patient from being disillusioned after trying to raise his/her urine pH and not getting anywhere. A simple key is when the pH readings vary greatly on arising each morning, It is almost certain that anxiety is influencing the individual's physiology.

Chapter 16

1 Wilkes D et al, *Medicine and Science in Sports and Exercise* 1983;15(4):277–280

2 Costill DL et al *Int J Sports Med* 1984;5:225–231

3 Sutton JR et al *ClinSci* 1981; 61:331–338. Rupp JC et al *Med and Sci in Sports and Exer* 1983; 15–115, McKenzie DC, et al *J Sports Sciences* 1986; 4:35–38

4 Mainwood GW et al *Canadian Journal of Pharmacology* 1980;58:624–632

5 Inbar O et al *J Sports Sciences* 1983; 1:95–104, Horswill CA et al *Med and Sci In Sports and Exer* 1988; 20(6):556–569. George KP et al ERGONOMICS 1983;31(11): 1639–1645

6 McNaughton LR, Cedaro R *The Aust Journal of Sci and Med in Sport* 1991; 23(3): 66–69

7 Old fashioned sodium bicarbonate baths for the treatment of psoriasis in the era of futuristic biologics: An old ally to be rescued; *Journal of Dermatological Treatment;* Volume 16, Number 1/February 2005

Chapter 17

1 http://emedicine.medscape.com/article/243160-overview

2 Russell RM, Golner BB, Krasinski SD, et al. "Effect of antacid and H2 receptor antagonists on the intestinal absorption of folic acid." *J Lab Clin Med* 1988;112:458–63.

Chapter 18

1 Bamberger and Avron 1975 *Plant Physiol* 56: 481–485

2 Ma J, Folsom AR, Melnick SL, Eckfeldt JH, Sharrett AR, Nabulsi AA, Hutchinson RG, Metcalf PA: Associations of serum and dietary magnesium with cardiovascular disease, hypertension, diabetes, insulin, and carotid wall thickness: the ARIC study. *J Clin Epidemiol* 48:927–940, 1985

3 Rosolova H, Mayer O Jr, Reaven GM: Insulin-mediated glucose disposal is decreased in normal subjects with relatively low plasma magnesium concentrations. *Metabolism* 49:418–420, 2000[Medline]

4 Resnick LM, Gupta RK, Gruenspan H, Alderman MH, Laragh JH: Hypertension and peripheral insulin resistance: possible mediating role of intracellular free magnesium. *Am J Hypertens* 3:373–379, 1990[Medline]

5 *Am J Physiol Renal Physiol* 243: F197-F203, 1982; 0363–6127/82

6 Bamberger and Avron 1975 *Plant Physiol* 56: 481–485

7 Effect of sodium chloride- and sodium bicarbonate-rich mineral water on blood pressure and metabolic parameters in elderly normotensive individuals: a randomized double-blind crossover trial. *J Hypertens.* 1996 Jan;14(1):131–5. Department of Internal Medicine, Universitatsklinikum Benjamin Franklin, Free University of Berlin, Germany.

8 www.amazon.com/Dietary-Reference-Phosphorus-MagnesiumFluoride/dp/0309063507/ref=sr_11_1?ie=UTF8&qid=1227893156&sr=11–1

9Biochem J. 1977 August 1; 165(2): 355–365. www.pubmedcentral.nih.gov/articleren-der.fcgi?artid=1164908

10 *Am J Physiol Renal Physiol* 243: F197-F203, 1982; 0363–6127/82

11 Origin of the Bicarbonate Stimulation of Torpedo Electric Organ Synaptic Vesicle ATPase. Joan E. Rothlein 1 Stanley M. Parsons. Department of Chemistry and the Marine Science Institute, University of California, Santa Barbara, Santa Barbara, California, U.S.A.

12 The method consists of using one tablespoon of magnesium carbonate to be dissolved with soda water. Buy a bottle of Carbonated Seltzer water - no sodium, just carbonated "fizz" water, unflavored. Refrigerate for a couple of hours. Get another, larger bottle, and pour 2/3 of a capful of plain (no-flavor) Philips Milk of Magnesia (which is Magnesium Oxide, an alkaline laxative) into the large bottle. (The bottle comes with a plastic measuring cup which is what I mean when I say 2/3 capful.) Now quickly open the bottle of carbonated water (water + carbonic acid) and empty it into the large bottle containing the 2/3 capful of Magnesia. Shake well. You will have a bottle of milky/cloudy liquid which is in the process of neutralization between the carbonic acid and the magnesium oxide—leaving a neutral salt, Magnesium Bicarbonate.

13 Perry, 1986; Perry and Laurent, 1990; Henry and Heming, 1998http://www3.inter-science.wiley.com/journal/119558225/abstract?CRETRY=1&SRETRY=0#c1

14 Forster and Steen, 1968; Maren and Swenson, 1980

15 Bamberger and Avron 1975 *Plant Physiol* 56: 481–485

16 "Regulation of Chloroplastic Carbonic Anhydrase." Effect of Magnesium, Michael A. Porter and Bernard Grodzinski. *Plant Physiology*, Vol. 72, No. 3 (Jul., 1983), pp. 604–605 (article consists of 2 pages) Published by: American Society of Plant Biologists

17 Mg^{2+} is critical for all of the energetics of the cells because it is absolutely required that Mg^{2+} be bound (chelated) by ATP (adenosine triphosphate), the central high energy compound of the body. ATP without Mg^{2+} bound cannot create the energy normally used by specific enzymes of the body to make protein, DNA, RNA, transport sodium or potassium or calcium in and out of cells, nor to phosphorylate proteins in response to hormone signals, etc. In fact, ATP without enough Mg^{2+} is non-functional and leads to cell death. Bound Mg^{2+} holds the triphosphate in the correct stereochemical position so that it can interact with ATP using enzymes and the Mg^{2+} also polarizes the phosphate backbone so that the 'backside of the phosphorous' is more positive and susceptible to attack by nucleophilic agents such as hydroxide ion or other negatively charged compounds. Bottom line, Mg^{2+} at critical concentrations is essential to life," says Dr. Boyd Haley who asserts strongly that, "All detoxification mechanisms have as the bases of the energy required to remove a toxicant the need for Mg-ATP to drive the process. There is nothing done in the body that does not use energy and without Mg^{2+} this energy can neither be made nor used." Detoxification of carcinogenic chemical poisons is essential for people want to avoid the ravages of cancer. The importance of magnesium in cancer prevention should not be underestimated.

18 Magnesium has a central regulatory role in the cell cycle including that of affecting transphorylation and DNA synthesis, has been proposed as the controller of cell growth, rather than calcium. It is postulated that Mg++ controls the timing of spindle and chromosome cycles by changes in intracellular concentration during the cell cycle. Magne-

sium levels fall as cells enlarge until they reach a level that allows for spindle formation. Mg influx then causes spindle breakdown and cell division.

19 Altura BM, Altura BT, "Role of magnesium in patho-physiological process and the clinical utility of magnesium ion selective electrodes." *Scand J Clin Lab Invest Suppl*, vol. 224, pp.211–234, 1996

20 "Influence of Bicarbonate Calcium-Rich Alkaline Mineral Water on Kidney Parameters in Comparison with Tabriz Tap Water in Patients with Renal Lithiasis." Department of Drug Applied Research Center, Tabriz University of Medical Sciences. Argani

21 Sebastian A, Harris ST, Ottaway JH, Todd KM, Morris RC Jr. "Improved mineral balance and skeletal metabolism in postmenopausal women treated with potassium bicarbonate." *N Engl J Med* 1994;330:1776–81

Chapter 19

1 *ClinicalPediatrics*, Vol. 23, No. 2, 94–96 (1984) DOI: 10.1177/000992288402300205

About the Author

Mark Sircus, Ac., OMD, DM (P) was trained in acupuncture and Oriental medicine at the Institute of Traditional Medicine in Santa Fe and the School of Traditional Medicine of New England in Boston. He also served at the Central Public Hospital of Pochutla, Mexico. He is part of the Scientific Advisory and Research Development team of the Da Vinci College of Holistic Medicine. Dr. Sircus' articles have appeared in numerous journals and magazines throughout the world. In addition, he is also the bestselling author of several books including *Transdermal Magnesium Therapy.*

Index

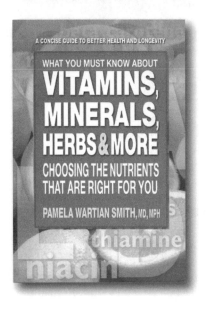

WHAT YOU MUST KNOW ABOUT VITAMINS, MINERALS, HERBS & MORE

Choosing the Nutrients
That Are Right for You

Pamela Wartian Smith, MD, MPH

Almost 75 percent of your health and life expectancy is based on lifestyle, environment, and nutrition. Yet even if you follow a healthful diet, you are probably not getting all the nutrients you need to prevent disease. In *What You Must Know About Vitamins, Minerals, Herbs & More*, Dr. Pamela Smith explains how to determine which nutrients are right for you, and how nutrient deficiencies can lead to chronic disease.

Part 1 of this easy-to-use guide provides the individual nutrients necessary for good health. In Part 2, it offers personalized nutritional programs for people with a wide variety of illnesses and disorders. People without prior medical problems—men, women, vegetarians, smokers, dieters, and more—can look to Part 3 for their supplementation plans.

Whether you want to maintain good health or are trying to overcome a medical condition, *What You Must Know About Vitamins, Minerals, Herbs & More* can help you make the best choices for your diet and supplementation program.

$15.95 US • 448 pages • 6 x 9-inch quality paperback • ISBN 978-0-7570-0233-5

SUICIDE BY SUGAR

A Startling Look at Our #1 National Addiction

Nancy Appleton, PhD, and G.N. Jacobs

More than two decades ago, Nancy Appleton's *Lick the Sugar Habit* exposed the health dangers of America's high-sugar diet. Now, in *Suicide by Sugar,* Appleton, along with journalist G.N. Jacobs, presents a broader view of the problems caused by our favorite ingredient. The authors offer startling facts linking a range of disorders, from obesity and cancer to our growing sugar addiction. Rounding out the book is a sound diet plan along with a number of recipes for sweet, easy-to-prepare dishes made without sugar.

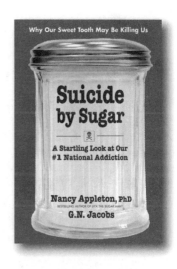

$15.95 US • 192 pages • 6 x 9-inch quality paperback • ISBN 978-0-7570-0306-6

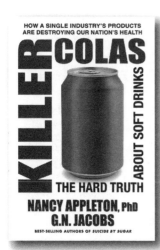

KILLER COLAS

The Hard Truth About Soft Drinks

Nancy Appleton, PhD, and G.N. Jacobs

Over the last few decades, the sale of sodas and sports drinks has exploded, as has the incidence of obesity, diabetes, hypertension, heart disease, cancer, and stroke. *Killer Colas* looks at the history and growth of the soft drink industry, explores its powerful influence over the media, and examines the harmful ingredients that these companies include in their formulas. It also offers scientific evidence that links America's consumption of soft drinks with our declining health.

$15.95 US • 144 pages • 6 x 9-inch quality paperback • ISBN 978-0-7570-0341-7

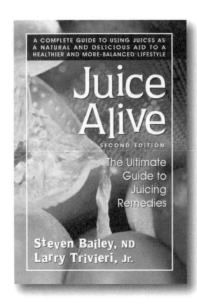

JUICE ALIVE,
SECOND EDITION
The Ultimate Guide to Juicing Remedies

Steven Bailey, ND and Larry Trivieri, Jr.

It's a fact—the juice of fresh fruits and vegetables provides a powerhouse of antioxidants, vitamins, minerals, and enzymes. With just a single glass of juice daily, you can heal, nourish, and protect your body safely and naturally. The trick, of course, is knowing which juices can best serve your individual needs. In this interesting and easy-to-use guide, health experts Dr. Steven Bailey and Larry Trivieri, Jr. tell you everything you need to know to maximize the benefits and tastes of juice.

The book begins with a unique look at the long and fascinating history of juicing, from Hippocrates to hip juice bars. It then examines the many components that make fresh juice truly good for you--good for weight loss, for renewed energy, for mental clarity, and for so much more. Next, it offers practical advice about the various types of juices available, as well as buying and storing tips for fruits, veggies, and herbs. The second half of the book begins with an important chart that matches up a host of ailments with the most appropriate juices. This is followed by over 100 delicious juice recipes. Also included is a juice cleansing regime and beauty program.

If you've never juiced before, let *Juice Alive* introduce you to a world bursting with the exciting tastes and incomparable benefits of fresh juices.

$14.95 US • 288 pages • 6 x 9-inch quality paperback • ISBN 978-0-7570-0266-3

**For more information about our books,
visit our website at www.squareonepublishers.com**